anaesthesia under examination

 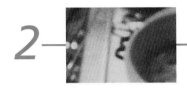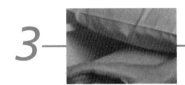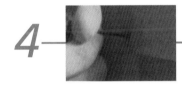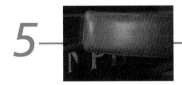

Contents

© Audit Commission 1997

First published in December 1997 by the Audit Commission for Local Authorities and the National Health Service in England and Wales, 1 Vincent Square, London SW1P 2PN

Printed in the UK for the Audit Commission by Belmont Press.

ISBN 1 86240 060 1

Photographs: David Mansell (Cover, pp33, 12, 17, 28, 40, 54, 58, 74, 88, 91, 103) with thanks to Northwick Park Hospital, Emap Elan (p78).

Illustration: Fred Van Deelen, p5.

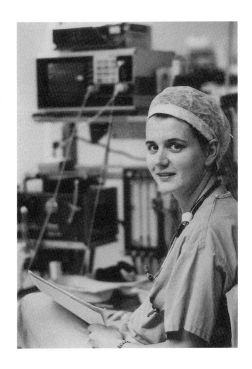

Preface

Few mainstream medical specialties are understood as little as anaesthesia. Yet without anaesthesia services and modern pain control, most surgery cannot take place. Under a general anaesthetic the patient enters a complex, pain-free state – not merely sleep – when the function of many of the body's vital systems are modified and monitored carefully by the anaesthetist. And more and more patients are coming into contact with anaesthetists outside the operating theatre. Some anaesthetists specialise in critical care, where longer contact makes them more familiar to patients and their relatives, and patients needing advanced forms of pain control after their operation often have their therapy monitored closely by an anaesthetist. Mothers requesting an epidural will have it administered by an anaesthetist, and people with long-lasting, intractable pain will often be cared for by an anaesthetist at a chronic pain clinic.

The Audit Commission chose this study because NHS trust chief executives voted it the most important topic during consultation. Anaesthetists are directly involved in the care of patients on whom two-thirds of acute trusts' income depends, and they are the biggest single group of doctors within every acute hospital. Trust managers, anxious to meet their surgical contracts, often express uncertainty about whether anaesthetists are as flexible as they might be, and are being deployed in the best possible ways. In response, anaesthetists point to hospitals with few surgical list cancellations caused by anaesthetists, to the long hours that many work, and remind trusts that they often manage theatres and day surgery units efficiently.

This is the context in which the study is set. The report explores whether anaesthetists truly limit trusts' ability to deliver their core services, and sets out good practice in how they can in fact enhance it. It considers the place of anaesthetists in a patient-focused hospital, and illustrates the problems that can arise when interdisciplinary teamworking breaks down, using the example of pain after surgery. Over the next year the Audit Commission's appointed auditors will be assessing where each local trust stands, and how services for patients can be improved.

The study was carried out by Dr Richard Waite, David Bawden and Lucy McCulloch, under the direction of Dr Jocelyn Cornwell and Dr Jonathan Boyce. Lara Bryant, Dawn Carrol, Emma Cox, Linda Jarrett, Angela Lane, Jo Marsh, Dr Henry McQuay, Mark Pilling and Paul Smith contributed directly as members of the study team or as consultants. Appendix 1 lists members of the advisory group, together with the NHS trusts that were visited or provided data during the study. The Audit Commission is grateful to them all. Responsibility for the contents and conclusions rests solely with the Audit Commission.

Introduction

What anaesthetists do

1. Anaesthetists are doctors whose clinical skills are used throughout the hospital [BOX A]. They specialise in anaesthesia,* which translates from the Greek as 'without feeling', and analgesia ('without pain'). Their knowledge is applied most frequently to allow surgeons to operate by changing patients' sense of feeling – on average 75 per cent of clinical time is spent supporting surgery. How quickly patients recover from their anaesthetic, and are relieved of postoperative pain and side-effects such as nausea and vomiting, has a crucial impact on the rates of day surgery and inpatient lengths of stay that a trust can attain. Developments in anaesthesia not only enable complex surgery to be carried out on patients previously considered to be too high risk, but they also drive efficiency improvements in trusts.

* There is a glossary of technical terms at the end of the report. Endnotes are also gathered together at the end of the report.

BOX A

Anaesthetists work throughout the hospital

Anaesthetists' special clinical skills are used throughout the hospital. They:

❶ are needed at all planned and emergency operations where a general anaesthetic is used, to allow surgery to take place (and administer most local anaesthetics also);

❷ advise on or are involved in the preparation of surgical patients and the relief of pain and side-effects afterwards;

❸ often take the lead in managing patients in intensive care units (ICU);

❹ play an important part when women are giving birth (for example, administering epidurals for pain relief, and providing anaesthesia at caesarean section operations);

❺ work with patients with long-standing debilitating pain (chronic pain management), and usually lead acute pain teams;

❻ play a major role in cardiac-arrest 'crash' teams;

❼ provide pain relief and anaesthesia for patients with major trauma in accident and emergency departments;

❽ sedate, ventilate or manage the airway of some patients undergoing radiology and radiotherapy procedures;

❾ provide anaesthesia and pain relief for some dental patients; and

❿ provide anaesthesia for psychiatric patients receiving electro-convulsive therapy (ECT).

BOX A (cont.)

Anaesthetists work throughout the hospital

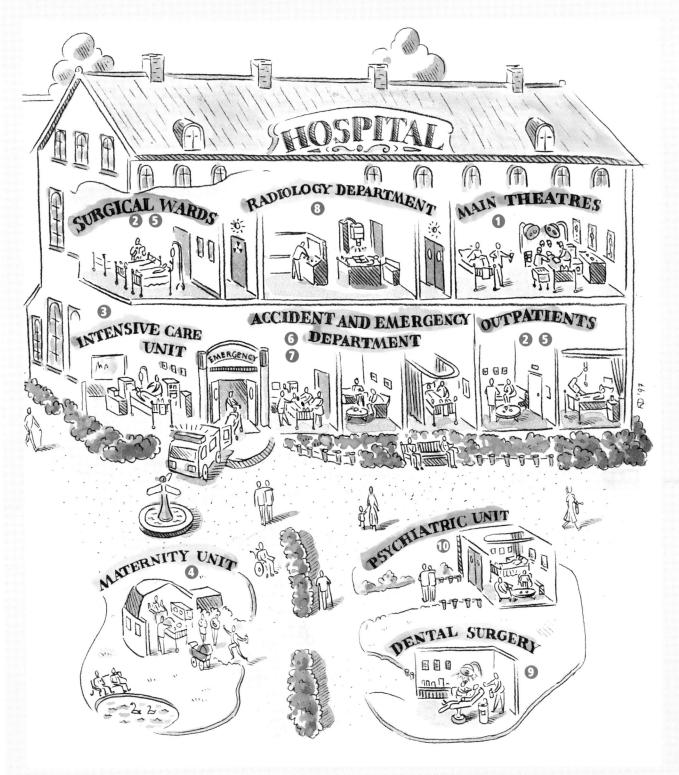

Source: Audit Commission, based mainly on publications by the Royal College of Anaesthetists and Association of Anaesthetists

2. This work involves a wide spectrum of difficulty. For example, when providing anaesthesia during thoracic or heart operations, the work can be complex and highly skilled because of the preparation and maintenance involved. For many routine operations the anaesthesia care is relatively standard. But the patient's medical condition, airway and other problems, can mean that inducing and maintaining a pain-free state for surgery is a risk to life, and call on an anaesthetist's diagnostic skills and experience. Anaesthetists' specialist knowledge of how to assist breathing, maintain cardiovascular, renal and liver function and ensure adequate replacement of blood and fluids also enables them to play a key role in treating emergency and intensive care patients. And their knowledge of anaesthetic and analgesic drugs allows them to play a specialist role in relieving the pain of both surgical and other patients.

3. The skills and attitudes of anaesthetists have a fundamental impact on the success of an acute trust. In 1995/96 in England and Wales the 5,500 anaesthetists of all grades (2,400 consultants)[1] were directly involved with two-thirds of patients, underpinning £10 billion of income at a pay cost equivalent to 3 per cent of this sum. In one small trust, anaesthetists' pay costs are the equivalent of 3.2 per cent of contract income; the £1 million spent on them directly underpins £21 million of patient care. In a large teaching hospital, pay costs of £4 million underpin £71 million [EXHIBIT 1].

EXHIBIT 1

Anaesthetists' pay costs in relation to the trust income that they directly affect

Anaesthetists have a key impact on two-thirds of an acute trust's income.

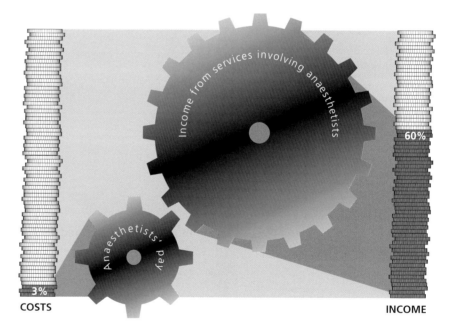

COSTS

INCOME

Source: Audit Commission study sites

The anaesthesia costs of a common operation

The two main components of cost are the anaesthetist and other staff who work in the operating theatre and look after patients recovering from the anaesthetic, and the equipment, drugs and consumables that the anaesthetist uses.

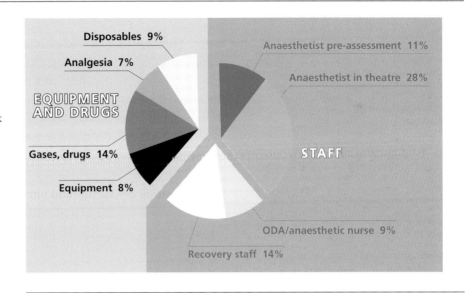

Source: Audit Commission, based on information reported by Broadway & Jones[2]

4. The three main types of doctor providing anaesthesia services are consultants, non-consultant career grades and trainees. These differ in the amount of training that they have successfully completed and their level of experience (the main sub-grades in the latter two categories are described in the glossary). In addition to doctors, the other two main components of the anaesthesia service are the operating department assistants (ODAs) and nurses who work in the operating theatre with the anaesthetist and look after patients recovering from an anaesthetic, and the equipment, drugs and consumables that anaesthetists use [**EXHIBIT 2**]. Added to these costs are those of the managers, secretarial support, training and other activities that an anaesthesia directorate needs or must carry out in order to provide patient services.

What the report aims to do

5. The Audit Commission's study, conducted between spring 1996 and summer 1997, considered value-for-money aspects of anaesthesia services in England and Wales. The study has confirmed that there are many good things about the current arrangements:

*   most anaesthetics – and all general anaesthetics given in hospitals – are provided by highly trained anaesthetists (or doctors in training);

*   UK anaesthesia has a world-class clinical, training and research reputation, with anaesthesia-related mortality reduced to very low levels;

*   most anaesthetists work long hours and are dedicated to providing a good service;

*   the Royal College of Anaesthetists and the Association of Anaesthetists have established standards and guidelines of good practice; and

*   in some trusts, anaesthetists take a leading role in the management of theatres, intensive care units and day surgery units to maximise operating efficiency.

6. But NHS trusts still face important challenges, and the intention of this report is to help to spread information about the good practice that exists. There is considerable variation in the organisation of anaesthesia services, beginning with a 15 per cent difference between the top and bottom quartiles in the staff costs of clinical sessions, and a 77 per cent difference between trusts at the extremes [EXHIBIT 3]. The report identifies what causes variations in costs and quality, and describes practical ways in which trusts can improve the provision of anaesthesia and pain relief services. Local audits will follow at each acute trust in England and Wales during 1998.

EXHIBIT 3

The annual cost* per session of anaesthetists' clinical work

There is a 15 per cent difference in staff costs between the top and bottom quartiles, and a 77 per cent cost difference between trusts at the extremes.

Annual medical staffing cost per scheduled clinical session (£000)

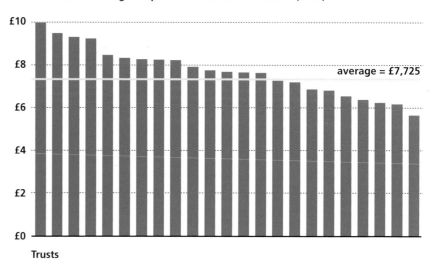

* Costs are calculated by dividing the basic salary costs of anaesthetists by the total number of clinical sessions that are regularly scheduled for anaesthetists in each trust. This includes normal weekday sessions in ICU and the maternity unit (ten sessions each if continual cover by one anaesthetist is provided). Anaesthetists also provide on-call services, administration, audit and training within these costs. Salary costs are the standard mid-point for each grade, to allow for easier comparison between trusts. Trainees have been included at 50 per cent of their salary costs because their time is split between training and providing a service contribution, and half of their costs are met via a central source of funding and not from trusts' clinical contract income. If trainees are included at 100 per cent, the average cost per clinical session rises to £8,900.

Source: Audit Commission, analyses of template rota and staffing establishments from 23 trusts (see Appendix 3 for more details)

7. The chapters explore the various components of costs (see the cost component tree and definitions in Appendix 3), showing even those trusts that are overall most economical where they can improve efficiency provide a better match of skills to needs and improve quality [EXHIBIT 4, overleaf]:

- In the face of rising costs and constant pressure to keep costs down and improve efficiency, **Chapter 1** considers how trusts can achieve the right number and mix of doctors, operating theatre staff and equipment – the building blocks of the service. The most important recommendations are aimed at meeting consultant shortages and making good the declining amount of service contribution that trainees can offer.

- **Chapters 2 and 3** examine day-to-day variation in costs and quality. Both chapters concentrate on anaesthesia services for surgical patients. Chapter 2 shows how trusts can plan a better match between the level of anaesthetists' skills and experience and patient needs, especially outside normal working hours. Many trusts can reduce costs by introducing new ways of providing flexible absence cover, already in use in a few.

- **Chapter 3** is about the quality of the information that surgical patients receive about their anaesthetic and how well their pain is relieved after surgery. Anaesthetists are justifiably proud of their role in developing acute pain services, but all trusts need to work continually to ensure effective collaboration between surgeons, anaesthetists and nurses – at the moment too many patients suffer pain after surgery because co-ordination is difficult to achieve. Written information needs to improve, and trusts need to recognise the importance of training ward nurses because they are best placed to monitor patients' changing pain levels.

- **Chapter 4** considers how trusts can decide on what makes a cost-effective mix of surgical and other anaesthesia services. Trusts vary greatly in the resources that they invest in maternity and chronic pain, without clear evidence about the effects on patient care. The recommendations call for anaesthetists, the trust board and purchasers to work together on defining service standards and the resources needed to deliver them. Nationally sponsored research is needed about the links between staffing levels, the number and type of patients, and outcomes.

- **Chapter 5** considers the management culture that is needed to foster the achievement of so many changes, and how these problems might be tackled in the longer term. Too little time is given to clinical directors in many cases, and in others frustration develops because they lack the power to make changes. Changing contractual arrangements may be the way forward, allowing for more flexibility in defining commitments than the present job plan allows, and linking this to the development of appraisal systems for individual consultants.

EXHIBIT 4

A map of the report

The chapters explore the various components of costs, showing even those trusts that are overall most economical where they can improve efficiency provide a better match of skills to needs and improve quality.

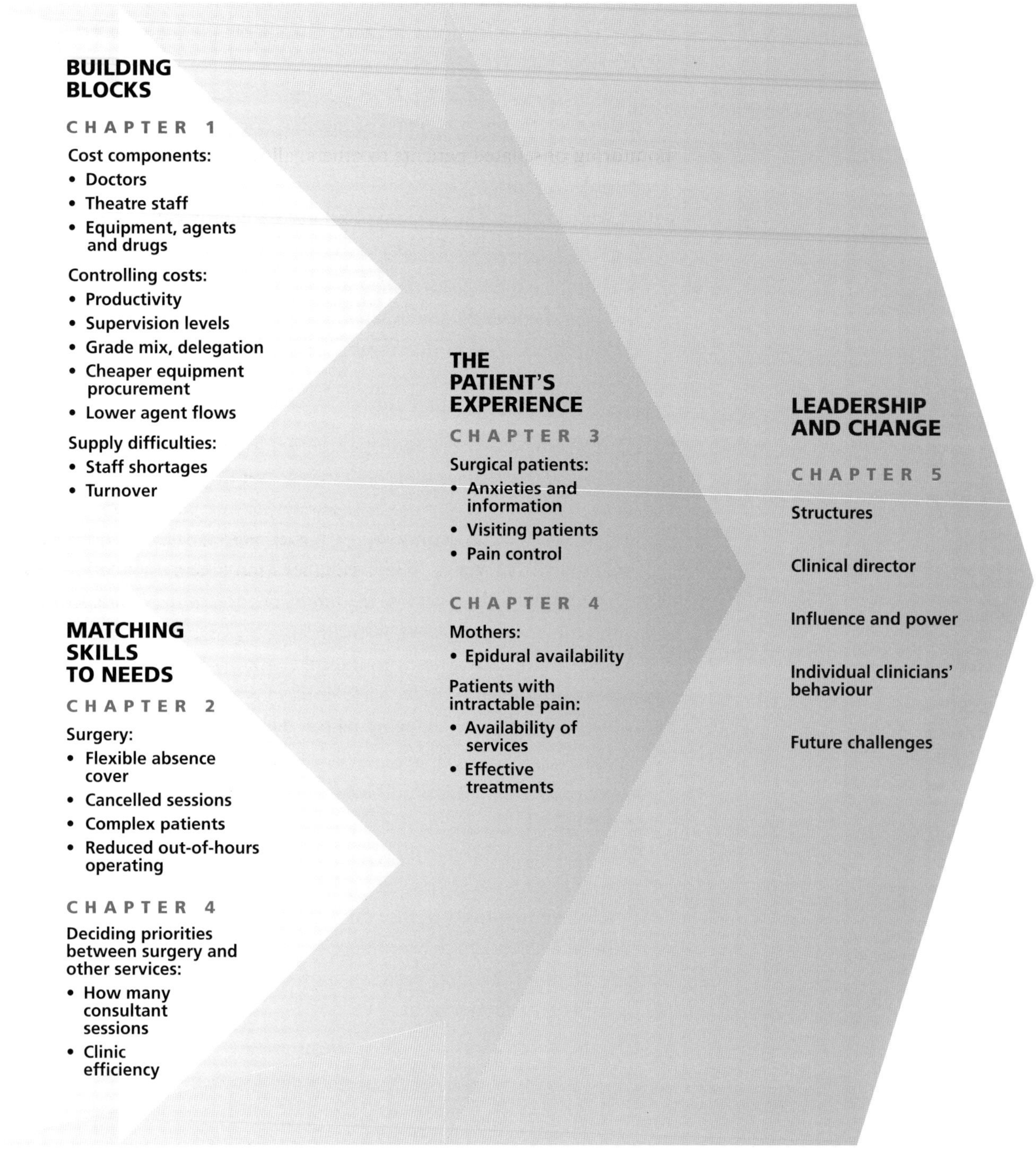

BUILDING BLOCKS

CHAPTER 1

Cost components:
- Doctors
- Theatre staff
- Equipment, agents and drugs

Controlling costs:
- Productivity
- Supervision levels
- Grade mix, delegation
- Cheaper equipment procurement
- Lower agent flows

Supply difficulties:
- Staff shortages
- Turnover

THE PATIENT'S EXPERIENCE

CHAPTER 3

Surgical patients:
- Anxieties and information
- Visiting patients
- Pain control

CHAPTER 4

Mothers:
- Epidural availability

Patients with intractable pain:
- Availability of services
- Effective treatments

LEADERSHIP AND CHANGE

CHAPTER 5

Structures

Clinical director

Influence and power

Individual clinicians' behaviour

Future challenges

MATCHING SKILLS TO NEEDS

CHAPTER 2

Surgery:
- Flexible absence cover
- Cancelled sessions
- Complex patients
- Reduced out-of-hours operating

CHAPTER 4

Deciding priorities between surgery and other services:
- How many consultant sessions
- Clinic efficiency

Source: Audit Commission

The practicability of change

8. There is little that trusts can do to avoid the cost increases caused by rising patient numbers and the reductions in trainee doctors' service contributions. However, within the current framework they can make efficiency improvements that will help to contain the rate of cost increases, improve the quality of patient care and manage the competing demands for anaesthetists in different areas of the hospital more effectively. There is also a way that might relieve the problem of finding enough doctors, and that might also reduce costs, that has yet to be tried in the UK. Anaesthesia in this country has evolved as a doctor-based service. It is high cost and high quality. By delegating some of the monitoring of sedated patients to others, allowing one anaesthetist to be responsible for two or more patients at once, more patients can be treated with fewer doctors. The staff involved are frequently called 'nurse anaesthetists', although they do not have to come from a wholly nursing background. Although common in some parts of the developed world, this system is the subject of strong professional opposition in the UK. Its potential to solve problems in the next millennium is discussed in the last chapter.

9. The details of the research on which this report is based can be found in Appendix 2. The main sources are national surveys of consultant shortages and acute pain services, detailed data collection at a randomly selected sample of over 40 trusts, and in-depth interviews with staff and patients at seven trusts representing the extremes of size and drawn from across England and Wales. While there are many recommendations for clinical directors and managers, the report is not just for 'management' – there are also good practice lessons that individual anaesthetists and nurses will wish to consider. Some of the issues go beyond the anaesthesia department – for example, the number of patients anaesthetised could be limited by a lack of beds for surgical patients, or for many other reasons outside the control of anaesthetists themselves. While the study has not gone into these areas in depth, they will require action at trust board and national levels.

1

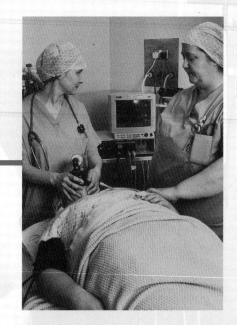

The Building Blocks of an Anaesthesia Service

Trusts are facing a rising demand for anaesthesia services at the same time as the service contributions of trainee doctors are declining. In the face of these pressures, trusts need to review the way that they deploy doctors, operating department assistants and nurses, and use equipment and drugs. Costs differ considerably due to variations in staffing levels, grade mix and the amount of supervision provided.

Introduction

10. Three building blocks make up the anaesthesia service – doctors, operating theatre and support staff, and the equipment and drugs used. Trusts can act to ease recruitment difficulties and employ an economical grade mix (while taking account of supervision and quality needs). They can also ensure that anaesthetists are contracted to deliver the maximum number of clinical sessions recommended under national terms, and that they have a staffing deployment plan (called a 'template rota') which maximises productivity. This chapter looks at ways in which medical staff can free up some of their time by delegating some tasks to others (in particular, the collection of patient test and case history information). It also comments on the use of theatre equipment and drugs.

Doctors

11. How many anaesthetists does a trust need? In a sense the answer is straightforward for surgery, because current ways of working require, for the most part, one anaesthetist to be present for every surgical session that a trust chooses to carry out.[3] Deciding on doctor numbers is more difficult in the other areas in which anaesthetists work, and Chapter 4 is about the scope that trusts have for changing and improving the ways that they provide two key services – for mothers and for patients with chronic pain. Further problems lie in deciding on the right grade mix, in translating the number scheduled to work every day into an establishment that takes account of training and supervision needs and absences, and in finding and retaining staff in a competitive employment market.

Rising costs

The number of consultant anaesthetists employed by NHS trusts increased by 41 per cent between 1986 and 1996

12. One of the key difficulties facing trusts is that the cost of employing doctors is rising all the time. This means that trusts must frequently review how many staff they need, and may find recruitment difficult. The number of consultant anaesthetists employed by NHS trusts increased by 41 per cent between 1986 and 1996 (Ref. 1). This rate of growth has been faster than that for surgeons (36 per cent), even though trusts recruit less than a whole-time equivalent anaesthetist to cover the operating lists created by the appointment of each new surgeon.[4] The faster rise in the numbers of anaesthetists is often attributed to the amount of non-surgical work that anaesthetists do – for example, in ICU, maternity units, chronic pain clinics and in management tasks. The second main driver is the reduction in the service contribution of trainee doctors.

13. The rise in numbers of anaesthetists is expected to continue. National planning models have been geared to supply enough trainees to allow a growth in the number of consultants of 5 per cent each year, because:

- **There is more work to be done:** for example, more patients are having operations,[5] more mothers are having their babies by caesarean section and are having epidurals for pain relief in normal labour, more emergency patients are being admitted, more patients are being treated in intensive care units.

- **Changed grade mix:** national planning aimed to double the number of consultant anaesthetists between 1988 and 2002, as part of a process

Locally, trusts need to review all aspects of anaesthetist employment and deployment to contain current rates of the increase in costs

common to all specialties following the recommendations of the national *Achieving A Balance* document (Ref. 2).

- **Reduced service contribution by trainee doctors:** the 'New Deal' limits the number of weekly hours worked by a trainee doctor to 56, and the new specialist training scheme (Calman) does not allow middle-grade trainees to work as many solo sessions, covering for absent consultants, if they are to complete training within the allotted time (Refs. 3, 4, 5).[6] More doctors will be needed to deliver the same amount of clinical work. For example, at one large hospital the number of operating sessions provided solo by trainee doctors halved between 1994 and 1996; since trainees were covering one-quarter of all sessions, and career grade staff three-quarters, the latter must now cover 12 per cent more sessions, or sessions must be cancelled. This will be an important cost driver over the next few years because although by March 1997 80 per cent of trainee posts met the New Deal target,[7] few trusts have worked out how best to meet the long-term reduction in service contributions from each cause.

- **More management:** consultant anaesthetists are taking part in directorate management and assuming the management of theatres and day surgery units.

14. The speed of the rise in anaesthetist costs prompts important questions about whether the NHS can afford to sustain this rate of increase, and whether enough new anaesthetists can be supplied year after year. The increase in anaesthetist posts needed can be dramatic for individual trusts – for example, at one hospital a fundamental review of workloads by the medical director and clinical director for anaesthesia suggested a need to increase in one year the number of consultant posts by one-third, and the number of non-consultant career grade doctors by half.

15. There needs to be national debate on how to face the future. But, locally, trusts need to review all aspects of anaesthetist employment and deployment to contain current rates of the increase in costs. The next three sections consider the main components of anaesthesia costs that they can influence:

- staffing levels and productivity (individual workloads, the actual hours worked by anaesthetists and the costs of providing supervision);

- grade mix; and

- the cost of making good consultant shortages.

Staffing levels and productivity

16. Anaesthetist staffing levels vary between trusts – some employ nearly 50 per cent more staff than others to deliver the same number of clinical sessions [EXHIBIT 5A], and the number of half-days in the week devoted to the different kinds of work – for example, surgery, other anaesthesia services and management – varies [EXHIBIT 5B]. While casemix differences mean that some trusts have a higher proportion of lists that need two anaesthetists for safety or efficiency reasons, casemix cannot explain the degree of variation shown in Exhibit 5. There are three more likely reasons:

- absence rates and how absence is covered (dealt with in Chapter 2);

- individual anaesthetist productivity – variations in the amount of care that each anaesthetist provides in the different clinical areas; and

- variations in the amount of 'doubling up' for training and supervision purposes.

EXHIBIT 5A

The clinical productivity of anaesthesia departments

Anaesthetist staffing levels vary between trusts – some employ nearly 50 per cent more staff than others to deliver the same number of clinical sessions.

Clinical sessions scheduled each week

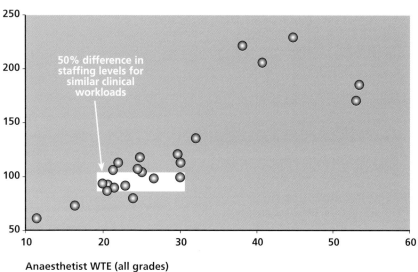

Anaesthetist WTE (all grades)

EXHIBIT 5B

The number of half-days* in the week devoted to fixed commitments – for example, surgery, other** anaesthesia services and management – also varies.

Average number of half-days for fixed commitments per WTE consultant anaesthetist

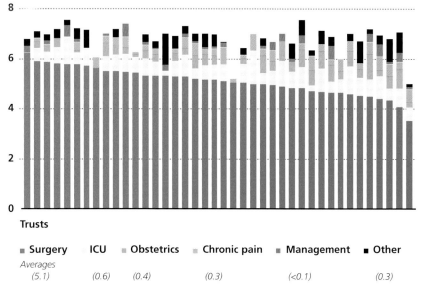

Trusts

■ Surgery	ICU	■ Obstetrics	■ Chronic pain	■ Management	■ Other
Averages (5.1)	(0.6)	(0.4)	(0.3)	(<0.1)	(0.3)

* Consultants' contracts are specified in terms of 'notional half-days' (NHDs) lasting 3.5 hours each.

** 'Other' includes radiology, acute pain, ECT, specific teaching duties.

Source: (A) Audit Commission analyses of template rota and staffing establishments from 23 trusts; (B) Audit Commission data request for job plan information, results for 40 trusts; definitions in Appendix 3

Most consultants have seven or more half-days for fixed commitments in their job plans, making their contracted clinical workload as high as expected under national terms and conditions – but one-quarter have fewer

Individual workloads

17. A consultant employed under national terms and conditions of service should have a job plan specifying the amount of time in a normal week to be spent on different commitments. The guideline is that consultants with whole-time or maximum part-time contracts should have a weekly work commitment equivalent to ten 'notional half-days' (10 x 3.5 hours), of which between five and seven should normally be 'fixed' commitments (Refs. 7, 8, 9, 10). Fixed commitments include operating lists, work in the maternity and intensive care units, pain relief clinics and other clinical work, plus specific management or similar duties. The flexible commitments that make up the remainder of the contract include all other activities undertaken by consultants on behalf of the NHS, including pre- and postoperative care of patients, emergency on-call, training and administration.

18. On average, fewer than 0.1 fixed commitments are assigned to management duties, since most consultants do not have any fixed commitment allowance for management duties, while a few (for example, clinical directors) have one or more. Differences between trusts in time allowed for management have only a small effect on the average number of clinical commitments in job plans (Exhibit 5b; management issues are picked up again in Chapter 5). Nevertheless, it is important for the next analysis to exclude clinical directors, part-timers, and other consultants who might be expected to have a reduced number of clinical commitments. The number of half-days devoted on average to *clinical* work per consultant anaesthetist can then be compared [**EXHIBIT 6**]:

- most consultants have seven or more half-days for fixed commitments in their job plans, making their contracted clinical workload as high as expected under national terms and conditions – but one-quarter have fewer; and

- trusts vary in how they handle clinical commitments – of 36 trusts, 15 have written a consistent number of half-days for fixed clinical commitments into the job plans of all their anaesthetists (12 trusts have all their anaesthetists with seven half-days for fixed commitments, two have all their anaesthetists with six, and one trust contracts for five) while other trusts have a mixture.

EXHIBIT 6

Variation in the number of
half-days for clinical work
per consultant anaesthetist

Most consultants have seven or
more half-days for clinical fixed
commitments in their job plans,
but one-quarter have fewer, with
considerable variation between
trusts.

Note: Bar sizes represent the percentage
of consultants with each number of
fixed commitments.

*Source: Audit Commission, results for
368 consultants in 36 trusts; excludes
anaesthetists with non-clinical fixed
commitments*

Number of fixed commitments for clinical work

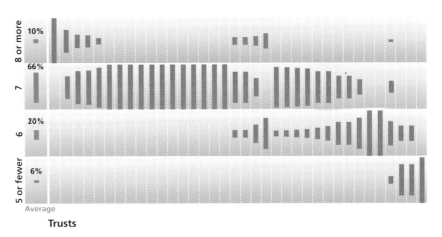

Trusts

19. If consultants have fewer than seven half-days for clinical
commitments, it should be because some other aspect of work is more
demanding than average. One obvious contender is the amount of on-call
work. We assigned consultants to three different groups according to how
often they are on-call (for example, one in every four nights, one in every
eight, etc), how many calls for advice they report receiving when on-call,
and how often they go into the hospital. On average, consultants with the
heaviest on-call workload are more likely to have a reduced number of
half-days for fixed commitments.[8] But the relationship is weak – three of
every five consultants with intense on-call workload still have as high a
fixed workload as others and, contrary to what might be expected, a few
retain eight or more half-days for fixed commitments.

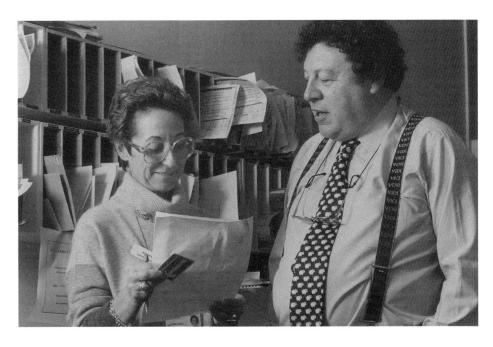

20. A further cause of variation is differences in the number of notional half-days that trusts allow an anaesthetist who is working an all-day operating list. Such operating lists for anaesthetists may extend beyond seven hours and, if a continuous cycle of preparing-monitoring-recovering is used to maximise throughput efficiency, they may not break for lunch. In these situations some trusts recognise an all-day list as two half-days in the anaesthetist's job plan, while some count it as three half-days. If the tendency for all-day operating lists continues to grow, this type of irregularity will cause noticeable differences in unit costs between trusts.

Actual hours worked by anaesthetists

21. Many anaesthetists who were interviewed or returned questionnaires commented on the long hours that they work. The exact relationship between contracted and rostered hours, and those actually worked in a week is not accurately known – trusts do not have the information that they need to assess workloads properly.[9] For this study consultant anaesthetists provided self-report estimates of the length of their last operating session, and actual work when on-call. There is considerable variation in individual workloads for reasons that include:

- Anaesthetists' actual operating session lengths vary from an hour (because the session was curtailed due to a lack of patients on the list, or some other event) through to nearly twice as long as the session time of 3.5 hours. Anaesthetists begin preparing patients before surgery commences, and stay to recover the last patient and ensure that pain relief has been initiated. For these reasons, operating session lengths are on average longer than the standard session length of 3.5 hours [**EXHIBIT 7**].

EXHIBIT 7

The actual length of anaesthetists' operating sessions

On average, anaesthetists' operating session lengths are longer than the standard session length of 3.5 hours because they prepare patients before surgery commences, and stay to recover the last patient and ensure that pain relief has been initiated.

Source: Audit Commission, self-reported timings for the most recent morning and afternoon lists of 413 consultants from 42 trusts

Anaesthetists' time from starting work in the anaesthetic room, to handing the last patient to recovery staff (in hours and minutes)

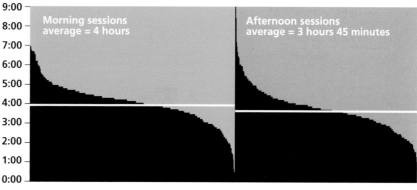

Morning sessions average = 4 hours

Afternoon sessions average = 3 hours 45 minutes

Consultant anaesthetists

- Anaesthetists spent an average of 40 minutes visiting patients before these lists took place (time which most trusts expect to come from the flexible element of job plans), with some doing no pre-visiting at all, and others spending over an hour (the quality effects of this variation are discussed in Chapter 3).

- The intrinsic difference between operating theatre sessions and sessions in ICU and maternity: in the latter, consultants do not have to find time for pre-visiting in their flexible sessions, but some report that training and emergency demands mean that they spend longer in ICU and the maternity unit than their sessional allowance.

- The number of telephone calls received at home when on-call varies by factors of several hundred per cent between doctors, and the hours spent in hospital show similar variation [EXHIBIT 8].

22. The consequences of these kinds of variations in contractual terms and hours worked are considerable. For example, anaesthetists with six half-days for clinical commitments are potentially offering 15 per cent less clinical work for their salary than those with seven. And those with seven or more, who also have very onerous on-call, teaching and management duties, may be working at a level that is not sustainable in the long term. This is neither a new problem, nor one unique to anaesthetists – it has already been pointed out by the Audit Commission in *The Doctor's Tale* (Ref. 9) – but some trusts still need to revise their consultants' job plans. Unless there are strong local reasons – for example, especially intense on-call – then all anaesthetists in a trust should be on seven half-days (or more where extra payment or other contractual agreement is in place).

EXHIBIT 8

The intensity of on-call duties

The number of hours spent in hospital when on-call varies between individuals by factors of several hundred per cent.

Source: Audit Commission, self-reported timings for the most recent weekday on-call of 516 consultants from 42 trusts

Hours spent in the hospital last weekday on-call

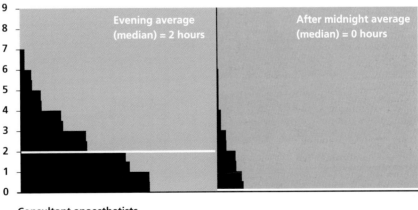

Evening average (median) = 2 hours

After midnight average (median) = 0 hours

Consultant anaesthetists

Research is needed to help trusts to calculate more accurately the number of consultant sessions needed both to produce well-trained anaesthetists and to meet the service requirement for surgery, intensive care, maternity and other services

23. A review of job plans is only a first step. Trusts also need to make sure that the mix of commitments matches purchasers' changing contract demands, and that job-plan commitments translate into a productive planned rota. There are some instances where consultants have seven half-days for fixed commitments in their job plan, but are rostered for only six, because an operating session has been cancelled in the long term. Coupled with differences in the actual time spent on duty, the result is differences in individual workloads and therefore overall trust productivity. Many consultants commented on these inequalities and the effects on both themselves and trust efficiency overall. Medical staff planning is taken up again in the final chapter.

Supervision costs

24. The cheapest short-term way to staff most sessions is to have individual anaesthetists working alone. But some complex cases need two pairs of hands, and a few operating sessions can be cost-effectively staffed by two anaesthetists because the gain in rapid turnover of patients through the theatre outweighs the extra staffing cost. In addition, directorates must provide trainees with opportunities to work alongside consultants. But trusts vary widely in the number of directly supervised sessions that are provided for trainees, and there is variation within trusts week by week [EXHIBIT 9] and for different grades. Despite the variation, most directorates provide trainees with direct supervision for more than half of their sessions. The result is that most sessions have more than one anaesthetist present – consultants, on average, work less than half of their sessions single-handedly.

25. The Royal College of Anaesthetists recommends that trusts provide a minimum of three sessions a week of direct supervision for each trainee, and that this guideline is used flexibly to meet local circumstances.[10] But it is unknown exactly how many are needed per week to meet the new 'Calman' training requirements. Because of the cost to trusts of 'doubling up', it is timely to estimate as accurately as possible the actual number of directly supervised sessions needed to produce each well-trained doctor via a structured training programme, replacing the input-based guideline. Research is needed to help trusts to calculate more accurately the number of consultant sessions needed both to produce well-trained anaesthetists and to meet the service requirement for surgery, intensive care, maternity and other services.

EXHIBIT 9

Direct supervision of trainees by consultants

Trusts vary widely in the number of directly supervised sessions provided for trainees, and there is variation within trusts week by week.*

* Each trust provided data for two to four sample weeks during 1996/97. Each square represents one sample week. The sample weeks for one trust are joined by a vertical line.

Source: Audit Commission, analyses of weekly rota from 24 trusts

Percentage of trainees' theatre sessions directly supervised by a consultant

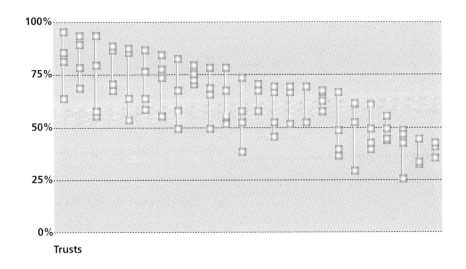

Trusts

Grade mix

26. The grade mix in anaesthesia is more expensive than for most other specialties, with more consultants and no house officers [**EXHIBIT 10**], mainly because the limited amount of ward work reduces the opportunities for using lower grades to carry out routine and less skilled work.[11]

EXHIBIT 10

Grade mix in anaesthesia compared with all hospital specialties

Anaesthesia contains more consultants than most other specialties, and no house officers.

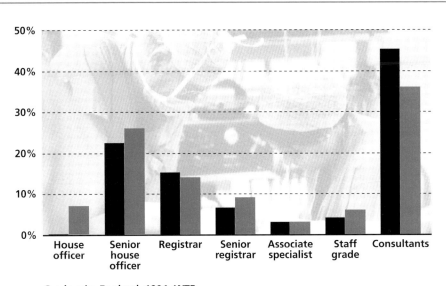

Grade mix, England, 1994, WTE

■ Anaesthesia   ■ All specialties

Source: NHS Executive medical staffing census September 1994; anaesthesia is compared with the average for all hospital specialties

27. Some trusts have higher costs than others, either because they have fewer trainee doctors, or because they employ fewer non-consultant career grade doctors – trusts vary from employing none to over one-third of such staff [EXHIBIT 11]. Furthermore, pay within the consultant grade can vary by 100 per cent, due to differences in pay points or distinction awards – in one trust, where the average of 12 consultants' salaries was £68,000, the range was from £50,000 to £105,000. If a trust has low turnover and a high proportion of long-serving, and eminent, anaesthetists, the costs of anaesthetising patients will be substantially more than in a department with mostly new, young consultants. Part of this cost is borne by the trust, and part centrally.

28. The most common of these non-consultant, non-training, grades are called 'associate specialist', 'staff grade' and 'clinical assistant'. One way to reduce cost pressures and make good the reducing amount of absence-cover offered by trainees is to increase the number of such staff. But while the number of consultant posts in anaesthesia has been rising faster than in most other specialties, new staff grade posts have grown at a slower rate. When these posts are advertised, the number of applicants has averaged 5 to 6 per post, compared with a rate for consultants of 1.4 per post, suggesting that a supply of people interested in this type of employment is available.[12] Until this year, the NHS Executive controlled the number of staff grades centrally (Ref. 13), although trusts have been free to create their own grades for longer.

EXHIBIT 11

Differences in anaesthetist grade mix between trusts

Some trusts have fewer trainee doctors, and employ fewer non-consultant career grade doctors – for example, trusts vary from employing no non-consultant career grades to over one-third of such staff.

Percentage of whole-time equivalent anaesthetists

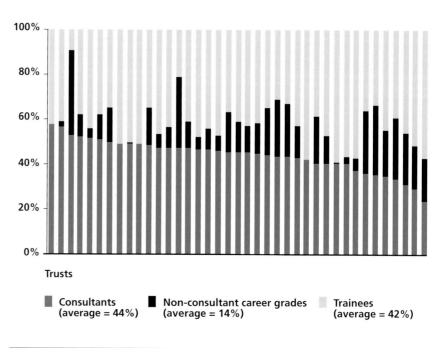

Trusts

■ Consultants (average = 44%)   ■ Non-consultant career grades (average = 14%)   ▪ Trainees (average = 42%)

Source: Whole-time equivalents, taken from budget statements from 39 trusts

TABLE 1

Anaesthesia qualifications of non-consultant career grade doctors

Qualification	%
FRCA – Part 3 or Final	32
FRCA – Part 2	25
FRCA – Part 1	6
FRCA – Primary	3
DA (UK) of the RCA; European Diploma of Anaesthesiology (or equivalent fellowships and diploma)	34

Source: replies to Audit Commission questionnaire from 106 non-consultant career grade anaesthetists in 40 trusts

29. If non-consultant career grades are employed, they should be deployed only for work appropriate to their level of skills and experience, which is variable [**TABLE 1**]. The difficulty for trusts trying to decide on an appropriate grade mix is that there is no research evidence to show whether trusts that employ higher numbers of non-consultant anaesthetists have different standards of patient care from those who employ fewer. Trusts should ensure that they audit the patient care of all grades of staff.

30. It is important that opportunities for continuing professional development (CPD) are made available[13] and the quality of the work of non-consultant career grade doctors is monitored and supervised by consultants as recommended by the Association of Anaesthetists (Ref. 14). Trusts vary considerably in the amount of direct supervision provided for these doctors, with one in five trusts providing none during the sample period [**EXHIBIT 12**]. In general, trusts providing the highest rates of supervision for trainees also tend to provide higher levels for other grades.[14] But with consultant time at a premium, some trusts concentrate on providing supervision for trainees, with non-training grades given a lower priority. And while the majority of non-consultant career grades report discussing their work in a formal one-to-one situation with a consultant at least once a year, one-third say this never happens. Only one in 20 reports having up-to-date written career development and training plans (N=106).

EXHIBIT 12

Direct supervision of non-consultant career grade anaesthetists by consultants

Trusts vary considerably in the amount of direct supervision provided for non-consultant career grade doctors, with one in five trusts providing none during the sample period.*

*Each trust provided data for two to four sample weeks during 1996/97. Each square shows the percentage of sessions supervised in one week. The sample weeks for one trust are joined by a vertical line.

Source: Audit Commission, analyses of weekly rota from 25 trusts

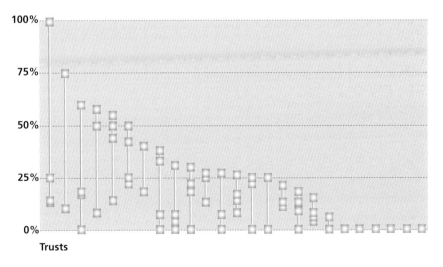

Percentage of non-consultant career grades' sessions directly supervised by a consultant

Consultant shortages

Two-thirds of trusts affected have been successful in solving their recruitment problems, but in some instances this has incurred extra costs

31. In a recent survey, anaesthesia was rated the acute-hospital specialty presenting trusts with most recruitment problems (Ref. 15). Shortages occur because demand has risen faster than recent national training supply, and because more anaesthetists are retiring early than the 3 per cent annually seen during the 1980s (Ref. 16). National action is increasing the number of available recruits for consultant posts, but the difficulty of predicting future demand makes it uncertain whether shortages will be completely solved (Ref. 17).

32. The majority (62 per cent) of trust personnel directors responding to an Audit Commission survey in summer 1997 said that their trust had experienced a shortage of consultant anaesthetists over the past five years. Most said that there had been little change over the years, but for 23 per cent recruitment had become easier and, for 16 per cent, harder. In summer 1997, half of trusts had full establishments, and one half had some vacant posts. On average, those trusts with shortages had 13 per cent of their funded establishment posts vacant (lower quartile 9 per cent, upper quartile 20 per cent).

33. Two-thirds of trusts affected say that they have been successful in solving their recruitment problems, but in some instances this has incurred extra costs. Trusts can improve their situation by paying closer attention to grade mix and the other cost-control mechanisms described in this and the next chapter, and by improving their recruitment and retention techniques [BOX B].

BOX B

Recruitment and retention

Trusts have tried to solve consultant shortages most commonly by increasing the number of non-consultant anaesthetists, and by enhanced compensation.

The most common short-term solution has been to 'throw money at the problem', by offering to pay consultants extra sessions or otherwise enhancing their remuneration package. One trust is paying some consultants for an eighth fixed commitment at an additional cost of £11,000 a year. Another has employed a consultant to do nine fixed sessions, with the extra two being paid at 2.5 times the NHS rate – coupled with increased advertisement effort, this trust turned a shortage of anaesthetists into a full complement within three years.

A longer-term solution is to ensure that existing doctors are working in the NHS – estimates across all specialties suggests that between one in five and one in ten doctors are not, often because they do not return after a career break to raise children (Ref. 18). Because a high proportion of the workload is fixed to the same time and day of the week, and with less continuing responsibility for patients, anaesthesia is a specialty that has attractions for

BOX B (cont.)

women doctors trying to combine working life with raising a family. The Royal College of Anaesthetists arranges special training programmes for doctors with family commitments who wish to train on a part-time basis. Nearly one-quarter of consultant anaesthetists are women, a higher proportion than the average for all hospital doctors, but some specialties have succeeded in attracting a higher percentage – for example, in paediatrics more than one-third of consultants are women. And the proportion of women in both anaesthesia consultant and training grades is growing more slowly than in the other main hospital specialties (Ref. 1). Anaesthesia should do more to promote the attractions of its working patterns to the increasing number of women entering medicine each year. Improvement is possible – in one trust, half of the consultant anaesthetists are women.

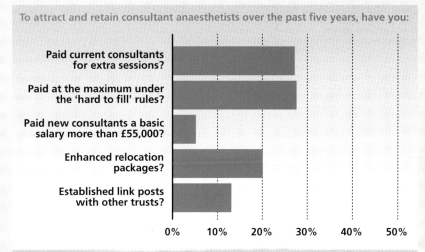

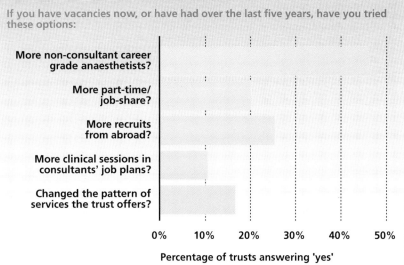

Source: Audit Commission, survey of trust directors of personnel; replies from 180 trusts

EXHIBIT 13

Consultant anaesthetist shortages across the country

The national picture is patchy without a clear geographical pattern to the distribution of vacancies.

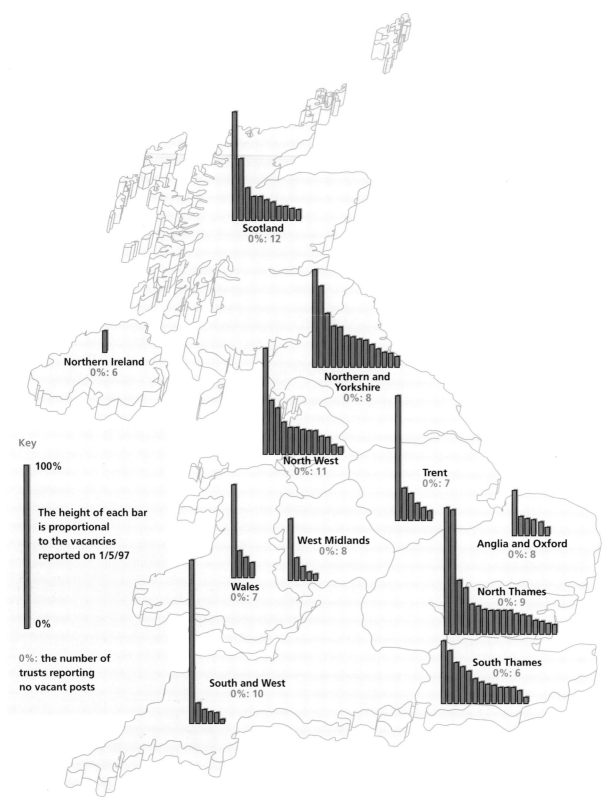

Key

100%

The height of each bar is proportional to the vacancies reported on 1/5/97

0%

0%: the number of trusts reporting no vacant posts

Scotland
0%: 12

Northern Ireland
0%: 6

Northern and Yorkshire
0%: 8

North West
0%: 11

Trent
0%: 7

Anglia and Oxford
0%: 8

West Midlands
0%: 8

Wales
0%: 7

North Thames
0%: 9

South Thames
0%: 6

South and West
0%: 10

Source: Audit Commission, survey of trust directors of personnel; replies from 181 trusts

34. The national picture is patchy [**EXHIBIT 13**]. Larger trusts – those with establishments of more than 15 consultants – are less likely to report vacant posts. In the worst cases – the 19 per cent of trusts which say that they have a shortage and have been unsuccessful in solving the problem – it becomes difficult to schedule enough operations and other elective work, such as normal labour epidurals for mothers or chronic pain clinics, and trusts lose contract income. The few consultants within these trusts carry more responsibilities – for example, in one trust the clinical director also takes the lead in several of the clinical specialties. They also work a more onerous on-call than in most other trusts, and must bear more of the training effort.

35. Trusts with consultant shortages pay high locum costs [**EXHIBIT 14**]. In the worst case, a trust with seven vacancies out of a consultant establishment of nine posts spends £265,000 a year on locums. In another trust, 20 per cent of the anaesthetists are agency locums, but they cost 25 per cent of total expenditure. To stay within budget the trust employs 17 per cent fewer whole-time equivalent doctors than it would if it had enough consultants in the establishment, largely because of extra on-call costs.

Other clinical staff

36. During surgery anaesthetists are supported by operating department assistants (ODAs). In a smaller number of hospitals, anaesthetic nurses undertake a similar role [**BOX C, overleaf**]. It is important not to confuse UK anaesthetic nurses with the nurse anaesthetists used in some other countries, who have a quite different role (see Chapter 5). The roles of staff in operating theatres have been changing over the last decade, but evidence is lacking to demonstrate improvements in either efficiency or effectiveness.

EXHIBIT 14

The cost of locum replacements for vacant consultant anaesthetist posts

Some trusts are paying high locum costs.

Source: Audit Commission, survey of trust directors of personnel; replies from 134 trusts

Total annual cost of locum consultant anaesthetists (£000)

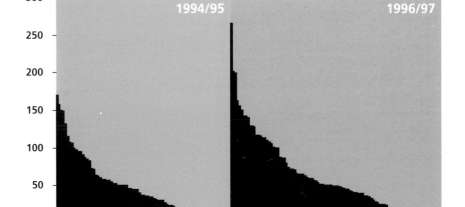

1994/95   1996/97

Trusts

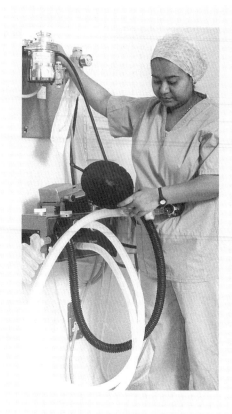

BOX C

Non-medical anaesthesia tasks in the UK

A second person – usually called ODA or anaesthetic nurse – is in most cases present with the anaesthetist in the operating theatre. These staff:

- assist the anaesthetist by checking and preparing the equipment and drugs that the anaesthetist will use, and attaching monitoring leads to the patient (such preparation might take five minutes for a straightforward day case patient, or up to an hour for complex patients);

- work with the anaesthetist during induction and arousal, including providing assistance in achieving vascular access and insertion of breathing tubes;

- may take some measurements during monitoring, and make sure the equipment continues to function properly during the operation;

- greet the patient in the anaesthetic room and play an important part in how patients react psychologically to their theatre experience; and

- outside the theatre suite, may take part in the hospital's cardiac-arrest team.

Flexible operating theatre staff

37. Traditionally, separate assistance for the anaesthetist and surgeon was the rule. 'Multi-skilling' – merging the previously separate roles of ODAs and anaesthetic, theatre and recovery nurses – was recommended by the 'Bevan' report on operating theatres (Ref. 19), and is supported by the Department of Health.[15] Most trusts have moved towards multi-skilling, but have normally involved only a minority of staff.

38. An important barrier to multi-skilling is that nurses and ODAs have separate basic training and qualifications. ODAs have a professional organisation that maintains a voluntary registration scheme and promotes standards of education and practice, but statutory registration is not required in the way that it is for nurses. While this remains the case, progress towards full multi-skilling will be hampered. It helps if trusts are explicit about roles and responsibilities. One trust has created teams consisting of a leader, and differing numbers of lead theatre practitioner, theatre practitioner and support worker. This structure paves the way for equal opportunities in career and personal development, since it is the competency of an individual to fulfil the role that is important, rather than whether they come from an ODA or nursing background.[16]

Extending the role of the anaesthetist's assistant in these ways does not offer cost-reduction opportunities, nor does it compensate for the reduced availability of trainee anaesthetists

39. The advantages proposed for multi-skilling include reduced absence costs and fewer session cancellations (because hospitals have a larger pool of staff to provide cover), and improved throughput efficiency. One hospital had a list cancellation rate of 7 per cent, similar to the national average at the time, but reduced this to 0.4 per cent after multi-skilling was introduced (Ref. 20). But the Audit Commission has found no consistent difference in cancellation rates between sites with differing numbers of multi-skilled staff, perhaps because of the difficulty of controlling for all the other possible reasons for cancellations.

Extended roles within the theatre suite

40. In addition to multi-skilling 'sideways', some staff have extended their roles 'upwards' to take on tasks traditionally undertaken only by doctors. For example, under the direct supervision of an anaesthetist, they may hand ventilate a patient, intubate, insert laryngeal masks, insert a cannula into the patient's arm and give intravenous drugs. But there is a lack of clarity about why such changes are taking place, and few trusts have written policies with stated objectives. As a recent NHS Executive-sponsored study concluded, the variation in who is doing what currently seen across the country demonstrates that there is scope for more systematic adjustment of roles (Ref. 21).

41. One of the main advantages of introducing surgical assistants, for example, has been to compensate in part for the reduced hours of trainee doctors – the assistants carry out work previously undertaken by a trainee doctor assisting the operating surgeon. But extending the role of the anaesthetist's assistant in these ways does not offer cost-reduction opportunities, nor does it compensate for the reduced availability of trainee anaesthetists, since it does not reduce the need for doctors. In fact, because higher skills and qualifications usually mean higher pay, it may increase costs still further. Research is needed to establish whether role extension can realise these potential advantages:

- faster throughput in theatre because the ODA or nurse can be doing a wider range of tasks while the anaesthetist is doing other things;
- allowing the anaesthetist to respond to an emergency while an extended-role ODA or nurse, who is able to some degree to understand what monitoring devices are telling about the patient's state, 'holds the fort' until another doctor arrives;
- enhanced operating theatre staff job satisfaction; and
- the ability to play a fuller role in the cardiac-arrest team, or in paramedic training.

Operating theatre staff costs

42. There is scope for savings in some trusts in operating theatre staffing levels and grade mix. A common pattern in the average theatre is to have three assistants, one of whom is dedicated to assisting the anaesthetist, plus a fourth who 'circulates' – for example, passing packs of equipment and dressings to the 'scrubbed', sterile members of staff. But some theatres also have a fifth member of staff undertaking miscellaneous duties and covering for meal breaks, and a few deploy a sixth for apparently similar casemixes. Trusts also differ in staff to patient ratios in recovery areas. In some cases, the higher staffing levels occur because of a complex casemix. But more often they reflect historical differences between trusts in the way that theatres are staffed.

43. In addition to staffing level differences, some trusts pay on average 25 per cent more per whole-time equivalent than others [**EXHIBIT 15**], because they employ fewer 'unqualified' staff (more accurately termed 'support staff' – average 18 per cent, but varying from nil to one-third) or have a higher grade mix among qualified staff. Trusts can achieve an economical grade mix by:

- deploying a support worker as one of the four staff per anaesthetic/operating room;

- rotating staff, rather than retaining highly graded staff on permanent nights, which attracts extra enhanced-hours payments; and

- relying on multi-skilled staff to allow theatres to run safely and efficiently with three rather than four staff on duty. Provided that the mix contains individuals trained to satisfactory levels in both anaesthetic and surgical assistance, the use of multi-skilled staff can offset the increased grade mix costs by reducing the number of staff.

EXHIBIT 15

Operating theatre grade mix costs

Some trusts pay on average 25 per cent more per whole-time equivalent than others because of more expensive grade mix.*

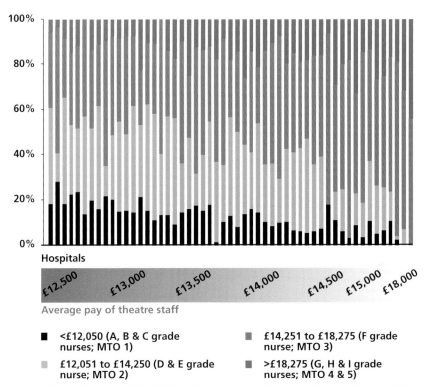

Percentage of whole-time equivalent theatre staff

Hospitals

£12,500 £13,000 £13,500 £14,000 £14,500 £15,000 £18,000

Average pay of theatre staff

- ■ <£12,050 (A, B & C grade nurses; MTO 1)
- £12,051 to £14,250 (D & E grade nurse; MTO 2)
- ■ £14,251 to £18,275 (F grade nurse; MTO 3)
- ■ >£18,275 (G, H & I grade nurses; MTO 4 & 5)

* Because some trusts no longer differentiate between ODAs and theatre nurses, the data provided here include all staff; further definition in Appendix 3.

Source: Audit Commission, analyses from 53 hospitals in 35 trusts

Delegation of preoperative patient preparation

44. Although trusts need to investigate further whether greater efficiency can be achieved by multi-skilling, extending roles and changing staffing levels within theatres, some trusts have eliminated tasks outside the theatre that do not make the best use of doctors' time. Anaesthetists need information about patients to decide if they are fit for surgery and, if not, what might be done to achieve fitness. If information-gathering is not done well, it can lead to inadequate assessment or cancellation of the operation. In some trusts the ordering of tests, and gathering of test results and case histories, is poorly organised. Forty per cent of consultant anaesthetists say that test results are often not available when needed, and 14 per cent had to spend time chasing these up themselves before their most recent list [**EXHIBIT 16A, EXHIBIT 16B**].

EXHIBIT 16A

Information the anaesthetist needs about the patient

In some trusts the ordering of tests or gathering of test results and case histories is poorly organised.

EXHIBIT 16B

Fourteen per cent of consultant anaesthetists said that they had to spend time in chasing up notes and ordering tests before their most recent list.*

* Information about patients on a consultant anaesthetist's most recent list could be provided by more than one means.

Source: Audit Commission study sites; 539 consultant anaesthetists' questionnaire replies from 45 trusts

Consultants reporting difficulties

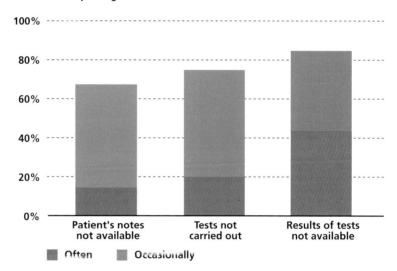

Tests and screening checklist gathered

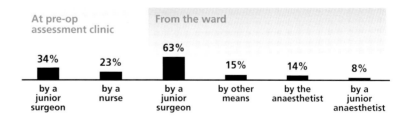

These measures reduce unnecessary stress for consultants and help to ensure that they can spend their time on work that makes the best use of their skills and experience

45. Gathering the information that anaesthetists need can be delegated without adverse effect. The key elements needed are:

- patient self-completion forms;

- nurse screening and testing; and

- agreements with the surgical teams about what standard tests anaesthetists always require.

46. Good collaboration between surgeons, anaesthetists, nurses and staff involved in handling admissions and waiting lists is needed if the process is to be efficient and effective:

- some surgical directorates invite anaesthetists to take part in the induction of new surgical trainee doctors;

- guidelines on anaesthesia requirements for preoperative tests can be inserted in surgical departments' handbooks, on surgical wards and in outpatient clinics;

- feedback from anaesthetists can be sought on over-testing, failure to test, and failure to have the results in time [CASE STUDY 1]; and

- the future emergence of pre-registration house officer (PRHO) posts that include an anaesthesia module, possible following recent changes to the regulations, could also facilitate collaboration.

47. If self-completion checklists for patients are introduced, it is important that the admitting nurse, trainee surgeon or anaesthetist does not then waste both the patient's and their own time by repeating the questions. The face-to-face interview should cover matters that cannot be assessed by questionnaire, tests and measurements, and include a discussion about the anaesthetic and pain control. In the future, patient-held computer-readable cards – or, in the interim, paper records – should be devised that can hold information about the patient's physiological state, previous operations, preferred analgesia and reactions to anaesthesia.

48. The principle of delegation also applies to nurses who set up patient-controlled analgesia in recovery, work in acute and chronic pain teams, and to midwives who top up epidurals. While these measures are unlikely to reduce the number of anaesthetists needed, they do reduce unnecessary stress for consultants and help to ensure that they can spend their time on work that makes the best use of their skills and experience.

Theatre equipment and drug costs

49. So far this chapter has shown that trusts vary widely in how efficiently they use the human resources that represent most of the cost of anaesthetising a patient. There is also variation in the remaining costs – equipment and drugs. Trusts can make savings via competitive tendering, standardising and bulk-buying, basing purchases on total lifetime costs, and making use of cost-efficient 'low-flow' methods of delivering anaesthetics.

CASE STUDY 1

Contrasting efficiency in pre-assessment processes

A. Operations cancelled on the day

At one hospital, anaesthetists are rarely involved with surgical patients until they receive operating lists, which typically arrive the day before the operating session. Anaesthetists cancel 1 per cent of operations. There are no agreed testing and information protocols between surgeons and anaesthetists, so information is patchy (for example, sickle cell testing may not have been carried out on at-risk patients), and little use is made of nurse- or patient-completed screening checklists. With better checks, anaesthetists believe that half of the anaesthesia-related cancellations could be prevented – for example, those patients arriving on the day of surgery with uncontrolled hypertension, or unmanaged diabetes symptoms.

B. Screening checklists

In a second hospital many admissions occur on the day of surgery, often as late substitutions. The introduction of pre-admission clinics on the wards, with a checklist provided for the admission nurses by the anaesthetists, and agreement on a protocol of tests that they wish the surgical team to carry out, has helped to make sure that anaesthetists have quick access to the information that they need. This is an economical system that is reported to work well.

C. Different information available in different specialties in the same hospital

In a third hospital, a protocol has been agreed with surgeons in one specialty, with the anaesthetist being called if results fall outside given ranges. With patients admitted in the morning of the day

before surgery there is time available for the anaesthetist to pre-visit all patients. On arrival at the ward, there is a package of test results waiting for the anaesthetist. Anaesthetists report favourably on the system and those nurses/trainee doctors providing the information. However, in a second specialty there are no agreed lists of tests, and screening is carried out variably – as a result, decisions about anaesthetic fitness are more problematic, and anaesthetists not always alerted when they should be. Also, test results are often not in the notes when the anaesthetist tries to find them – if results are not available on the day of surgery, then the patient is moved to the end of the list while results are awaited, or the operation is cancelled.

Equipment

50. Trusts should pay attention to the management of anaesthetic-related equipment for safety reasons and because of the scale of investment involved (for example, about £350,000 across all the theatres of one small trust, with the total for one operating theatre and anaesthetic room typically £50,000[17]). Professional guidelines recommend replacement about every decade (Ref. 22).[18] The Audit Commission has recently described how trusts can make savings by better procurement processes (Ref. 23), for example, by:

- economic ordering (aggregating purchases into one order whenever feasible, co-ordinating purchasing across the trust, buying only one product for each purpose, and evaluating between alternative products using total lifetime costs and not simply the purchase price);

- tendering both purchase and maintenance contracts; and

- developing a team approach to purchasing, bringing together the clinical, technical and procurement knowledge of an anaesthetist, an ODA, an engineer and a supplies officer.

In low-flow circuits, the amount of agent delivered can be reduced by capturing previously wasted agent in expired gas and recycling it

51. Anaesthetic rooms and theatres vary in how well equipped they are and in the age of equipment. Some trusts could make savings if they considered:

- reducing the number of spare machines;
- making one of the recovery ventilators transportable, for use around the theatre suite; and
- reducing the number of vaporisers to two, with a supply of a smaller number of vaporisers for other agents and spares held in reserve.

Drugs

52. The cost of anaesthetic drugs used in a medium-sized district general hospital with ten operating theatres is likely to be at least £300,000 a year. An important method of cost control is to ensure that a clinical and business case is always prepared for the inclusion of new drugs on the formulary. This should indicate the area and amount of use of the new drug, what drugs (if any) are being replaced, who will use the drug, clinical effectiveness and quality considerations, financial implications and funding. Most trusts have a Drugs and Therapeutics Committee to review proposals for new drugs to be included in the hospital formulary. This should be an appropriate forum to consider business cases, in addition to considering the clinical acceptability of new drugs. An example of such a process has recently been described (Ref. 24).

53. If new anaesthetic drugs are accepted on the basis that their area of use will be restricted, the anaesthesia directorate should have a plan for introducing and using the drug that will help to ensure its use in accordance with the agreed limitations. The plan should include guidelines on appropriate use of the drug, restrict access to the drug in anaesthetic rooms and to certain operating theatres, describe arrangements to monitor its use and how audit will assess whether the intended quality and cost benefits have been achieved.

Low-flow anaesthesia

54. A way of saving on the cost of anaesthesia without compromising patient care or safety is to invest in equipment that allows a reduction in the amount of agent used. In conventional inhalation anaesthesia using semi-open circuits, patients use only about 10 per cent of the agent, with the rest breathed out unused and wasted. In low-flow circuits, the amount of agent delivered can be reduced by capturing previously wasted agent in expired gas and recycling it. Very low flows are achievable by a few experienced anaesthetists at the cutting edge of these developments. But the majority of anaesthetists could safely operate flows of about two litres if the operating theatre has the necessary equipment. Typically, more than half of costs can be saved when flows are reduced to such levels.

55. On average, two-thirds of operating theatres are equipped for low-flow anaesthesia [**EXHIBIT 17**]. While nearly one-third of trusts have equipped all their theatres in this way, the remainder vary considerably. The investment payback period is one to two years, after which the potential annual saving for the remaining eight years of the equipment lifespan amounts to £850,000 across this sample of 25 under-equipped trusts (a conservative estimate based on flows recorded in a published case study (Ref. 25)). While these sums represent a small percentage of the total spend on the anaesthesia service in a trust, they are nevertheless worth realising.

56. Whether the theoretical savings are realised depends on anaesthetists using the equipment properly to achieve low flows. At two trusts surveyed where all operating theatres are already fully equipped for low-flow anaesthesia, expenditure on anaesthetic agents could be reduced by 18 per cent (£9,000) at one and 29 per cent (£11,000) at the other if all anaesthetists achieve flows of two litres a minute. Some anaesthetists will do better than this, so increasing the potential for savings.

57. This is a developing field of research for anaesthetists, with the potential for substantial economies in the future. Directorates need to make sure that they have guidelines on how to use the new equipment, and that training ensures that everyone is able to achieve low flows. This point leads on to the next two chapters – even if trusts are able to solve this chapter's problems and get the structure right, they are only part way to making sure that they are providing an efficient and effective anaesthesia service. Efficiency and quality problems can arise that are independent of the number of anaesthetists employed, but depend on how efficiently individuals work within those structures.

EXHIBIT 17

Savings from introducing low-flow circuits

In low-flow circuits, the amount of agent delivered can be reduced safely to about one-third of usual levels. On average, two-thirds of operating theatres are so equipped; across this sample of trusts, £850,000 a year could be saved if all invested in the equipment.

Source: Audit Commission study sites, 411 operating rooms in 36 trusts; definitions in Appendix 3

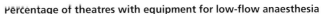

Percentage of theatres with equipment for low-flow anaesthesia

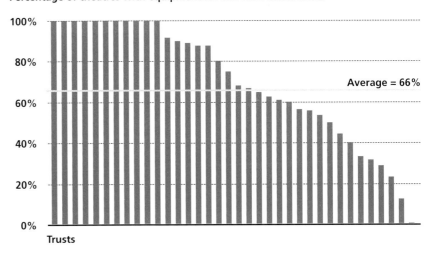

Average = 66%

Trusts

RECOMMENDATIONS

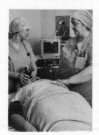

1 The Building Blocks of an Anaesthesia Service

The recommendations follow the order in which they are discussed in the text. Priority recommendations are highlighted.

Doctors

Detailed discussion and recommendations related to training and supervision, grade mix, recruitment and retention strategies, and medical staff planning have been made previously by the Audit Commission in relation to all hospital specialties (Refs. 9, 10). The recommendations given here should be seen as additional to those in the earlier reports, or as deserving particular emphasis in relation to anaesthesia.

	Recommendation	Action needed by
1	Agree explicit rules for calculating half-days for fixed commitments, and translate them into a written job plan for each consultant.	**Chief executive, medical director, clinical director**
2	Employ consultants on contracts with seven half-days for 'fixed'* commitments, a high proportion of which should be directly clinical, unless there are clear reasons why this is not appropriate for a particular trust or individual.	**Chief executive, medical director, clinical director**
	*Review the use of the term 'fixed', since it is good practice if some of these are used flexibly to cover for absent colleagues.	**NHS Executive**
3	Translate job plan commitments into a template rota that matches the trust's contract and patient care needs; review the template periodically to ensure that it continues to match these needs and adjust job plans as required (at least annually).	**Chief executive, medical director, clinical director**
4	Review periodically the actual hours worked by each consultant to ensure reasonable equality of workload across the trust, and high overall productivity.	**Chief executive, medical director, clinical director**

RECOMMENDATIONS

	Recommendation	Action needed by
5	Review whether the number of flexible, part-time trainee posts already available will be sufficient to maintain anaesthesia's attractiveness to the increasing proportion of women doctors emerging from medical schools.	**Personnel director, clinical director, postgraduate dean, Royal College of Anaesthetists**
6	Review grade mix, especially considering whether an increase in non-consultant career grades is appropriate for lists that have been covered in the past by trainees.	**Medical director, clinical director**
7	Agree a policy for the continuing professional development of non-consultant career grade doctors.	**Clinical director**
8	Link each non-consultant career grade doctor with a named consultant who is responsible for checking the quality of their work periodically and ensuring their access to direct supervision and training opportunities.	**Clinical director**
9	Sponsor research to determine whether the flexible 'three supervised sessions per week' recommendation can be replaced by guidelines that help trusts to calculate more precisely the number required to produce each well-trained anaesthetist, while providing as economical a way of staffing clinical sessions as possible.	**Royal College of Anaesthetists, NHS Executive, clinical directors**

Extended roles within the theatre suite

10	Agree a policy that sets out the reasons for extending the roles of ODAs or anaesthetic nurses (for example, extra safety, contribution to cardiac-arrest team, quicker theatre throughput).	**Clinical director, director of nursing, senior ODA, theatre manager**

RECOMMENDATIONS

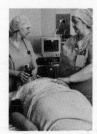

1   The Building Blocks of an Anaesthesia Service

Operating theatre staff costs

	Recommendation	Action needed by
11	Check grade-mix costs and reasons (for example, high grades on permanent nights, low use of unqualified staff); if it is policy to employ a highly qualified mix, then check that benefits such as quicker theatre throughput are being realised.	**Clinical director, theatre manager**

Delegation of preoperative patient preparation

12	Agree and issue checklists for completion by patients and/or nurse before admission, to help ensure that the necessary information is available for the anaesthetist in advance of surgery, and to avoid wasting expensive doctor time.	**Clinical director, director of nursing**
13	In the longer term, develop patient-held computer-readable cards – or, in the interim, paper records – for holding information not only about the patient's physiological state, but also about previous operations, preferred analgesia and reactions to anaesthesia.	**NHS Executive, trust chief executives**
14	Agree on the standard tests needed for different types of patient; effective collaboration is required to ensure that the necessary information is available for the anaesthetist when needed.	**Clinical directors of anaesthesia and surgical specialties**
15	Where patients are admitted on the day of surgery (whether day case or inpatient), pre-admission visits/clinics are a good idea for both information-gathering, and for giving the patient information and reducing anxiety.	**Medical director, surgical clinical directors**

RECOMMENDATIONS

Equipment and drugs

	Recommendation	Action needed by
16	If not already done so, review equipment procurement processes in line with the good practice described by the Audit Commission in *Goods For Your Health* (HMSO, London, 1996).	**Chief executive, clinical director**
17	Draw up a business case for the introduction of new anaesthetic drugs or agents which shows the costs of new against old, the benefits of the new, and gives guidelines of when using the new drug will improve costs or outcome. Introduce an audit system to evaluate whether expectations are met.	**Clinical director, head pharmacist**
18	Invest in low-flow equipment, and ensure via education and audit that low lows are achieved, and that the expected financial benefits ensue.	**Chief executive, clinical director**

2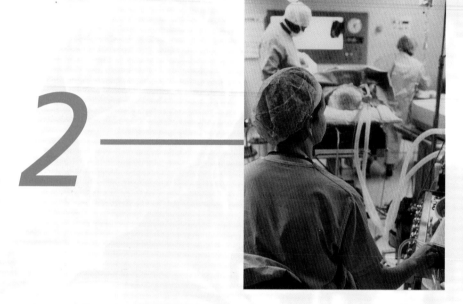

Matching Skills to Surgical Patients' Needs

On average, only a small proportion of operating sessions are cancelled because no cover is available for an absent anaesthetist. On paper, most theatre sessions have a consultant's name written against them, but legitimate absence means that one-third of planned consultant sessions (as well as most out-of-hours care) are provided by less senior doctors. Arrangements for cover in some trusts are better, and are based on guidelines and formal agreements.

Introduction

58. Trusts must match anaesthesia resources to the varying needs of patients while keeping costs as low as possible. The philosophy in some trusts is to provide a 'consultant-based' service, where a consultant is assigned to most of the planned clinical sessions. Consultant anaesthetists usually have a regular weekly timetable working with a small number of consultant surgeons. In this way, the anaesthetist and the surgeon work as a highly specialised partnership and know and understand each other well. However, legitimate consultant absences mean that these partners will not always work together – other consultants and other grades will provide some of the service, and the way that such absences are covered is of critical importance to quality and costs.

59. If clinical sessions are cancelled a trust could lose contract income,[19] and the higher the level of absence, the higher the cost of providing cover to avoid cancellations. Quality might also suffer because patients who are planned to be anaesthetised by a consultant do not benefit from that level of skill. Consultant shortages and a lessening of trainee doctors' service contributions could make these problems worse. This chapter shows the variation between trusts in the extent of these problems, and considers ways in which the effects can be mitigated.

Absence

60. Substantial legitimate absence for consultants is built into the system – with study, professional and annual leave allowances, each consultant is entitled to be absent for 15 to 20 per cent of the time. Operating theatre staff have less study leave, but sickness absence can be a problem.

Consultant absence

61. Most trusts draw up a template rota that shows the clinical sessions regularly provided by anaesthetists on each day of the week throughout the year, including out-of-hours emergency cover (discussed further in Appendix 3). On average, three-quarters of daytime sessions are planned to be covered by consultants – an apparently good response to the proposal in *Achieving A Balance* (Ref. 2) to increase the ratio of consultants to juniors. However, absence means that on average consultants attend only two-thirds of the planned sessions, and variation is high both between and within trusts [EXHIBIT 18, overleaf]. The result is that while the anaesthesia service has the appearance of being largely consultant-based, at least in normal weekday hours, the reality is often different.

EXHIBIT 18

The proportion of surgical sessions planned and actually provided by consultant anaesthetists

On average, three-quarters of surgical sessions are planned to be covered by consultants, but absence means that consultants attend only about two-thirds of the planned sessions.

Source: Audit Commission, analyses of template rota and weekly plans from 20 trusts

Percentage of surgical sessions at which consultant anaesthetists are present

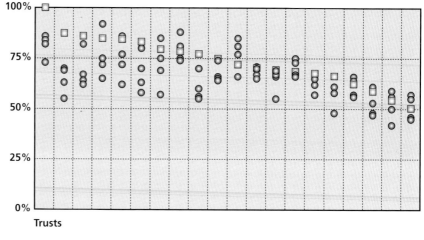

Trusts

☐ Planned cover
(average = 73 per cent)

○ Cover during four sample weeks
(average = 65 per cent)

Operating theatre staff turnover and absence

62. With operating theatre staff, turnover and sickness absence are the main cost contributors. While, on average, trusts lose 6 per cent of staff per year, one-quarter of trusts pay the recruitment, temporary cover and then induction costs for turnover rates that are two to three times greater. Similar differences exist for sickness absence costs – although, on average, absence per employee is six days per year, for some the cost is much higher. Most trusts spend less than 5 per cent of their costs on temporary agency or bank staff, but some incur the extra costs of a much higher proportion of such staff [EXHIBIT 19]. A further problem for trusts in certain areas of the country – mainly around London – is the cost of long-term use of agency ODAs to cover shortages. In one trust, nearly half the ODAs are long-term agency staff, costing the trust 1.7 times the usual base salary plus 25 per cent agency commission per whole-time equivalent.

EXHIBIT 19

Use of temporary staff in theatres

Most trusts spend less than 5 per cent of their costs on agency or bank staff, but some incur the extra costs of a much higher proportion of such staff.

Source: Audit Commission, analyses from 31 hospitals in 20 trusts; definitions in Appendix 3

Percentage of theatre staff from agency or bank

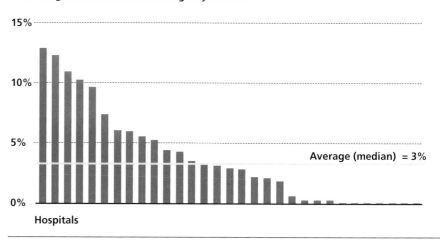

Average (median) = 3%

Hospitals

63. Geographical factors mean that some trusts can do little to avoid these costs. But trusts should ensure that they have examined the options available to control absence and turnover (for example, job enrichment schemes, career and educational opportunities and reviewing the salaries of establishment ODAs). General guidance on such personnel issues has recently been published by the Audit Commission (Ref. 26).

The cost and quality consequences

64. In addition to direct replacement costs, high absence levels cost more if they lead to clinical session cancellations. Absence may also produce a poorer match of skills to patients' needs, and have an adverse impact on the training needs of trainee anaesthetists.

Cancelled sessions

65. Cancellation of an entire operating session has a detrimental impact on the trust's ability to achieve surgical contracts. List cancellation rates vary from a few to nearly one-quarter – on average, only a small proportion of these cancellations occur because no cover is available for an absent anaesthetist [EXHIBIT 20], but in some trusts anaesthetist absence cover can become a major issue [CASE STUDY 2, overleaf]. It is important that trusts identify the real reasons for list cancellations – there are many possible causes apart from anaesthetists' absence. These include surgeon unavailability, insufficient patients to make up a list, lack of inpatient or critical care beds, and theatre or recovery staff shortfalls or absence (Appendix 4). Cancellations due to absent theatre staff are rare, but one-quarter of trusts stated that they are unable to schedule enough lists in the first place because of difficulties in recruiting staff.

EXHIBIT 20

The reasons for theatre session cancellations

Anaesthetists are responsible for only a small proportion of cancellations in most trusts.*

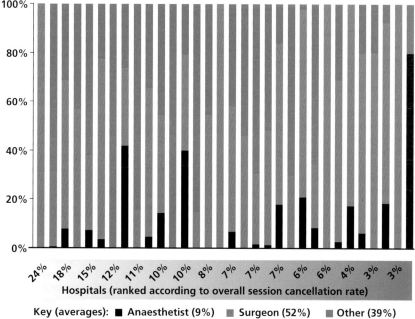

Percentage of theatre sessions cancelled

Hospitals (ranked according to overall session cancellation rate)

Key (averages): ■ Anaesthetist (9%) ■ Surgeon (52%) ■ Other (39%)

* Surgeons and anaesthetists usually cancel operating sessions for annual, study or professional duties leave, and audit sessions.

Source: Audit Commission, results from 32 hospitals in 30 trusts

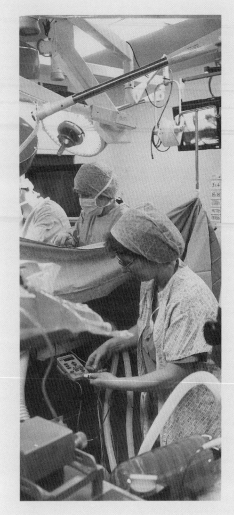

Theatre session cancellations by anaesthetists

In one hospital the rate of cancellations by anaesthetists doubled from a few per cent in 1994 to 5 per cent in 1996 and, on the basis of the first six months, looks set to double again in 1997. The directorate concerned believes that the reason is reduced cover available from middle grade trainees under 'Calman' requirements. It has yet to change its requirements on how consultants cover, or to appoint more non-consultant career grades, but it is actively considering the latter.

In another trust, the theatre department takes active steps to reduce cancellations caused by poor communications. It seeks out in advance likely cancellations due to anaesthetist or surgeon planned absence, and other foreseeable reasons. The revised timetable is published two weeks in advance, and the surgical specialties, anaesthesia department and theatre manager work together to re-schedule lists to avoid cancellations.

In a third trust, a system for 'selling' cancelled lists exists, with each surgical specialty keeping a close eye on the relationship between contract volumes and waiting lists. The opportunity for generating extra income, especially via GP fundholder cost-per-case contracts, exists. The number of cancelled sessions has reduced by half, because the cancelling specialty has a financial incentive to advertise its intention to cancel well in advance, and other specialties have a financial incentive to use available cancellations. While the anaesthesia department does not share in the financial incentives, the advance notice required by the system gives the department more time to plan replacement cover.

Complex patients and inexperienced anaesthetists

Each patient should be anaesthetised by someone with the experience and skills to match their needs

66. Each patient should be anaesthetised by someone with the experience and skills to match their needs, and the anaesthesia directorate's system of scheduling anaesthetists to clinical sessions should aim to achieve this match. But in some trusts, much of the least risky and routine planned work is done by consultants as part of their fixed commitments – as Exhibit 18 has shown, the proportion of sessions planned for consultant cover varies from 52 per cent to 98 per cent, a range unlikely to be explained by casemix differences.[20] Even if the planned rota does match skills to patients' needs, some complex patients may still be anaesthetised by trainee doctors either because surgery is performed at night when

consultants are on-call but not in the hospital, or during the day when trainees are covering for consultant absences (complexity is defined in Appendix 3). This raises questions about standards of care. Either complex patients anaesthetised out of hours by trainee doctors are receiving a poorer service than those who are attended by a consultant during the day; or patients anaesthetised during the day could receive good care without needing a consultant's level of skill.

67. The National Confidential Enquiry into Perioperative Deaths (NCEPOD) has shown that this mismatching of grades to patients' needs is a common problem. On average, half the patients who died around the time of their operation were anaesthetised by doctors below consultant grade, and nearly one in five by senior house officers (SHOs – the most junior of the anaesthesia trainees in most hospitals).[21] It is important to note that these patients could have died for many reasons, including their medical condition, that are quite unrelated to their anaesthesia. In Audit Commission study sites the pattern for all surgical patients, irrespective of their perioperative outcome, is the same. Data from the latter, more limited, sample of hospitals show that, while largely an out-of-hours problem, more patients are also anaesthetised by trainees within hours than most trusts would wish ([**EXHIBIT 21**] and earlier Audit Commission reports (Refs. 9, 32)).

EXHIBIT 21

Who anaesthetises patients?

While largely an out-of-hours problem, more patients are also anaesthetised by trainees within hours than most trusts would wish.

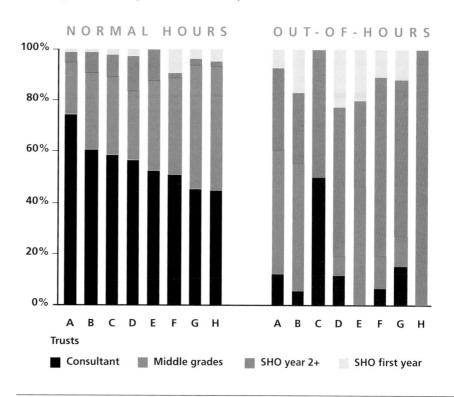

Percentage of different grades (most senior) present

Source: Audit Commission analyses of data collected by three-month (five trusts) or one-week (three trusts) surveys of surgical cases in study sites

Some trusts have introduced more flexibility into the way that absences are covered, and produce a better match of grade and experience of staff to patient need

68. Neither registrars nor SHOs should be alone when anaesthetising the most seriously ill of all patients (Refs. 27, 33). Since this issue was first raised by NCEPOD, the percentage of patients anaesthetised by these grades and classified as severely ill (ASA 4 or 5 – defined in the glossary) has declined steadily from 26 per cent to 19 per cent. Senior registrars have taken on more of these operations, while the percentage anaesthetised by consultants has remained steady at about 55 per cent. But the decline has been in the number of operations carried out by registrars. The percentage of such patients anaesthetised by the most junior grade – SHOs – has stayed steady at 6 to 8 per cent (Refs. 27-30).

69. There is a need for information that is more relevant to anaesthesia complexity than the ASA score, which is a measure of severity of illness. For this reason, the Audit Commission consulted with a number of anaesthetists to set out a method for categorising surgical patients by the difficulty and risk of anaesthesia (defined in Appendix 3). Initial results from eight trusts show that in each trust SHOs were the most senior anaesthetist at some operations classified as of high anaesthesia complexity. In each trust more complex operations are carried out at night than during the day, yet the grade mix of anaesthetists is more junior at night. These results suggest a need for research covering a longer sample period at more trusts. There are two aspects to this problem: first, how to ensure that trainees do not anaesthetise complex patients alone during normal hours on planned lists; and second, how to limit the amount of out-of-hours work despite rising numbers of emergency admissions.

Improvements

70. Some trusts have arrangements for cover that can reduce these cost and quality problems. They have introduced more flexibility into the way that absences are covered, and produce a better match of grade and experience of staff to patient need.

Control of absence entitlements

71. Some consultants are absent in excess of the 15 to 20 per cent expected because the trust has not made their entitlements clear. For example, some consultants count absent days and half-days as leave only when they have fixed sessions, and not on those days when they have no fixed sessions. Clear, written, rules and accurate records are needed [BOX D]. Senior doctors may be involved with regional, Royal College or other work of national importance that takes them away from their trust. There is no clear mechanism for compensating a trust for lost contract income because of these absences, nor for paying the trust to provide this expert advice.

BOX D

Good practice guidelines for managing annual, study and professional leave

- There should be guidance about how many anaesthetists can take leave at any one time.
- Fixed and flexible sessions lost through leave should roughly be in proportion to the number of each type of session.
- Days on which only flexible sessions occur should count as leave days if the consultant is away from the hospital and not contactable.
- Entitlement to days of leave in lieu should be stated clearly (for example, that days in lieu will not be allowed for bank holidays or weekends worked while on study leave).
- There should be prior notice sufficient to arrange cover.
- The clinical director should be informed of every absence from rostered sessions, and records of reasons should be kept for periodic review.
- Clinical directors should know about study leave taken in excess of the 30 days allowed over a three-year period so that they can decide whether it should continue and, if so, how it should be managed.
- Records of study and professional leave should be kept for all leave taken, not just that supported by the study leave budget.

Risk-sensitive cover systems for planned lists

72. It makes sense when covering absence to ensure that the most difficult sessions are covered by another consultant, and the less risky work by lower grades. Good communications should result in less complex patients being included in the operating list when the surgeon has been told in advance that a trainee will be providing absence cover for a consultant anaesthetist. Results from study sites show that six trusts did achieve such an appropriate casemix – on average, trainee anaesthetists in these trusts had a less complex casemix when covering for consultant absence than the average consultant casemix. But in two trusts this was not the case, and in two further trusts the casemix for trainees still included some patients classified as of high anaesthesia complexity.

73. A more formal system should produce a better match between casemix and grade. Clinical directors should grade operating lists and other kinds of patient activity by complexity, and then agree standards about which grade of anaesthetist is appropriate for each level of complexity. Formal systems of this type are rare [CASE STUDY 3]; usually, it is up to the rota planner or directorate secretary to match available names to slots that need cover as best they can. The system described in Case Study 3 is based on professional judgement, whereas what is needed is a research-derived method for classifying anaesthesia complexity. In the meantime, trusts can use the system described in Appendix 3 as a basis for regular audit of anaesthesia casemix in relation to grade of anaesthetist.

CASE STUDY 3

Providing standards-based cover

One hospital has devised a system that states the minimum level of anaesthetist considered safe to stand in for an absent colleague, based on professional judgement:

	Rota sessions
Session must be cancelled if consultant absent	9%
A consultant must provide cover	0%
Cover by at least an experienced specialist registrar (SpR3/4 or certain specified non-training grades)	21%
Cover by an SpR1/2	4%
Senior SHO	15%
Inducted SHO	8%
New SHO if a higher grade is immediately available	4%

Of about 170 sessions regularly scheduled on the template rota, 9 per cent are recommended for cancellation if the named consultant is absent. While some are specialist sessions where cancellation does reduce patient activity (for example, chronic pain management), most are sessions such as ICU, where on-call cover is of course still provided and patients are treated, but the extra knowledge and training offered by the regular consultant will be missing. Almost all the regular surgical sessions are rated as suitable for substitute cover.

None of the regularly scheduled surgical sessions is designated as needing another consultant to provide cross-cover, although this is the usual preference if one is available. This poses the question as to why the list is normally considered consultant-level. One reason is that temporary substitution by a lower grade is possible if the surgeon involved modifies the list to make sure that especially difficult cases are not called in for that session. It is not known how often during the year lists include such difficult cases and therefore need the consultant skills available to them on a regular basis, or whether critical incidents are more common during substitute-covered lists.

Source: Audit Commission site visit[22]

Most trusts should be able to cover a higher proportion of consultant absences by another consultant

Flexible absence cover by consultants

74. The grading of sessions just described allows more systematic planning for cover by subconsultant grades. But for both cost and quality reasons, it is better if consultants cover each other's absences. Many consultants already go out of their way to try to cover for absent colleagues, and resent suggestions that they are inflexible. But cover arrangements generally depend on good will, and can be a hit and miss affair. By adopting a more systematic approach to the problem, most trusts should be able to cover a higher proportion of consultant absences by another consultant.

75. It is the responsibility of the clinical director to ensure that services are covered. Methods exist for covering absence that can reduce cancelled sessions and allow risk-sensitive cover by different grades, but they are not used often enough [TABLE 2, overleaf]. The most important methods introduce more flexibility into cover by other consultants. Some consultants comment that flexible covering of other sessions on a regular basis is undesirable because the anaesthetist may be unfamiliar with the type of surgery, the way the surgeon works and the types of patient. But this must be balanced against the cost of otherwise cancelling a list, or having a more junior grade cover who will also be unfamiliar with the list.

76. While trusts will want to promote flexibility, they must be sensitive to the original contract of employment, and should ensure that the job content for which the consultant originally applied is not radically changed without agreement. And it can be difficult to change historical ways of working if there is a conflict between flexibility and fixed-time private practice arrangements. The level of flexibility depends on whether private practice is arranged as fixed pairings between surgeons and anaesthetists, or whether anaesthetists form a syndicate or consortium – the latter allows more flexibility when covering NHS absences, but is not within the control of NHS trusts. Trusts should employ new consultants on more flexible contracts that require absence cover across days, and should monitor sessions worked against contracted commitments so that consultants working under-commitment can cover absences.

Out-of-hours improvements

77. The most direct way to ensure that consultants provide emergency care would be to ask them to be in the hospital out of hours. But this would present problems in terms of quality of life for senior doctors,[23] and could be prohibitively expensive. At the moment consultants are expected to undertake on-call duties as part of their basic NHS salary and do not get paid extra if this entails coming into hospital. But this would no longer be the case if they were expected to be resident in hospital – currently agency locum anaesthetists must be paid to be on-call, and it typically costs the equivalent of a week's normal-hours salary for an agency locum to cover just one weekend.

TABLE 2

Varying degrees of flexibility in the arrangements for covering for consultants' absence

Cover arrangement used by all trusts

'Ad hoc' arrangements; consultants may cover absences on a voluntary basis. Similarly, trainees or non-consultant career grade staff are used to cover absences.

Cover arrangement used by some trusts	Often	Occasionally	Never
1. A group of consultants within one specialty provides internal cover for one another	12%	19%	69%
2. If their own session has been cancelled, and cover is needed at the same time, the consultant provides it	29%	68%	3%
3. If a session of their own has been cancelled, and cover is needed at any time within the same week, the consultant provides it	11%	51%	38%
4. If a session of their own is cancelled, the session is recorded as 'owed', and the consultant works an extra session either in the same week or in a future week when needed	11%	54%	35%
5. A consultant is re-allocated from their own planned session to cover for one that takes priority:			
– only if their own session goes ahead with trainee cover	10%	53%	37%
– even if their own session is cancelled as a result	–	24%	76%
6. Some consultants have one or more 'unallocated' fixed sessions in their job plans, used to cover absences:			
– they provide cover only on specific half-day slots	18%	27%	55%
– they cover if a cancellation occurs at any time of the week	–	25%	75%
7. Locum consultant employed	5%	45%	50%

TABLE 2 (cont.)

Other arrangements in use at individual visited trusts

- Non-consultant career grades have variable commitments and are mainly used to cover absence

- Trainees cover lists as part of planned solo experience

- Locum consultant employed only if other options are unavailable, and cost of otherwise cancelling session exceeds locum cost

- Sessions are ranked according to clinical and then contract value, and highest ranked lists are given priority when arranging cover for absences

- Specialties with the longest waiting lists are covered first.

Source: Audit Commission site visits, and questionnaire response from 38 trusts

Guidelines are needed that differentiate between true emergencies and patients whose operation can safely be deferred

78. Trusts should ensure that only genuine emergencies are operated on at night. On average, 15 per cent of patients are operated on outside scheduled sessions, but this varies from 3 to 25 per cent in different trusts. Guidelines are needed that differentiate between true emergencies (patients who must be operated on immediately because of the threat to 'life or limb') and those whose operation can safely be deferred to a scheduled daytime session, staffed by consultants [CASE STUDY 4, overleaf]. Reducing the number of operations carried out at night accords with recommendations made by NCEPOD. The decision to operate is a surgical one, but anaesthesia directorates need to ensure that subconsultant anaesthetists seek advice when complex patients arrive out-of-hours.

79. Trusts need to create theatre space for such sessions during the day – often called 'CEPOD sessions' because they are recommended by those reports – and make sure that they are properly staffed and not filled with extra elective patients. The most recent NCEPOD study finds that half of trusts have introduced at least one such daytime session (Ref. 31), but there are frequently problems with both anaesthetist and surgeon staffing – for example, not all trusts have anaesthetists with recognised commitments in their job plans to cover these lists on a regular basis.[24] But some trusts have been able to recruit new consultants with two daytime urgent/emergency sessions as part of their fixed commitment, who are attracted by the diversity and challenge of this type of work.

CASE STUDY 4

Reducing out-of-hours emergency operating

Trusts commonly use the NCEPOD classification of patients into emergency (immediate treatment) and urgent (treatment within 24 hours). One trust introduced another category, by classifying those needing immediate treatment separately from those needing treatment within 4, rather than 24, hours. This increased sensitivity reduced the number classified as emergencies by two-thirds, potentially allowing even more of those patients arriving after midnight to have their operations safely postponed until normal hours. But when actual practice was audited, the trust found that although 85 per cent of operations would have been suitable for postponement until normal hours, 76 per cent of operations were still being done out-of-hours. Ways of ensuring improvement are being discussed.

Another trust's guidelines state that consultants should anaesthetise at daytime emergency operations, and specialist registrars at operations between 5pm and midnight. While an SHO is first on-call after that, there are guidelines about the type of patient that they should anaesthetise without calling for more experienced back-up. Tightened rules about operating only on true emergencies after midnight mean that, on average, only one patient is anaesthetised in this large hospital per night when the first on-call is an SHO.

Consultants should take active responsibility for ensuring that more trainee and non-consultant career grade doctors follow procedures designed to deliver a safe service

80. NCEPOD reports that SHOs at half of the operations that led to perioperative deaths sought advice (Ref. 30). At some trusts, consultants expect trainees and non-consultant career grades to call them for advice or to come into the hospital, and there are guidelines stating when this is appropriate. But these guidelines are not widespread, and there are problems with compliance:

- 20 per cent of anaesthetists who responded to a recent survey about the effects of NCEPOD reports mentioned the introduction of local guidelines that match the grade of anaesthetist to case complexity (Ref. 36);

- fewer than one-third of trainees returning Audit Commission questionnaires knew of guidelines in their trust (replies from 362 trainees across 43 trusts), and few directorates systematically audit whether doctors actually follow the guidelines; and

- some trusts schedule a more senior anaesthetist to be in the hospital betweem 5pm and 9.30pm.

81. Consultants should take active responsibility for ensuring that more trainee and non-consultant career grade doctors follow procedures designed to deliver a safe service [BOX E].

BOX E

Proactive on-call

A proactive on-call system is one where senior anaesthetists take active steps to ensure that other doctors follow procedures and deliver a safe anaesthesia service out of normal hours. Trusts should ask themselves:

Are there guidelines about which grades are allowed to anaesthetise patients of differing complexity and risk?

Are there guidelines about when a doctor must seek more senior advice?

Has compliance with guidelines been audited? Did:

* doctors seek advice for cases where the guidelines said they should do so?

* consultants review case complexity?

* consultants actively encourage telephone calls for advice?

What happens if guidelines have not been followed? Is there a mechanism for ensuring compliance?

A consultant-led service

82. Many trusts assume from job plans and the template rota that their service is consultant-based, because most clinical sessions have a consultant's name written against them. But consultant absence means that on average one-third of planned sessions, and most out-of-hours care, is in fact provided by trainees or non-consultant grades. This raises important questions about the extent to which a consultant-based service is realistically achievable, or whether the NHS could afford it. It would:

* be expensive to employ enough consultants to cover all absence by that grade;

* deny some consultants the chance to specialise; and

* reduce training opportunities to an extent that the new shorter training periods might not be achieved.

83. While a consultant-based service may not be realistic, a consultant-led service is achievable. Trusts should decide on the quality standards that they wish to reach, and agree which sessions must be consultant-provided at all times, according to the difficulty of the lists. By formalising the cover rules and having a few consultants with one or two variable sessions, quality standards can be maintained without a substantial increase in costs.

84. The demands of shorter training periods, introduced by the Calman reforms, mean that trainees will be unable to carry out as much solo work if they are to gain the necessary supervised training experience in the time allowed. In addition, when they do have time to offer solo cover the restricted time they now have to become experienced in each subspecialty (typically, about three months) will make them less flexible in

offering to work in other areas. Finally, because they now train in each subspecialty for a shorter period, they will be less able to provide safe, experienced cover for the more complex lists. Thus, the burden for cover must fall more and more on non-consultant career grades recruited specially for the task and on consultants.

85. This chapter has shown how systems and resource levels can affect quality. But some of the problems for patients do not concern the number of anaesthetists available, or their grades, but are caused by how anaesthetists and other staff behave. Solutions involve doctors and nurses changing the way that they do things. Most of these changes are resource-neutral and mean that trusts can make significant improvements for the better. This is the subject of the next chapter.

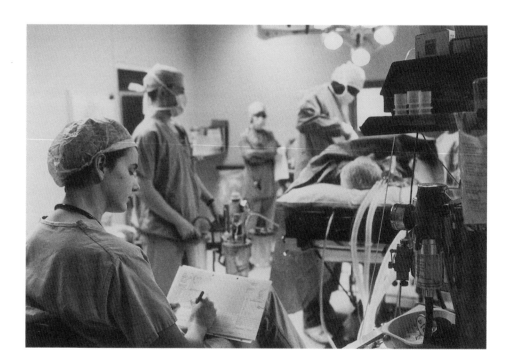

RECOMMENDATIONS

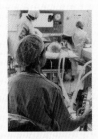

2 ── Matching Skills to Surgical Patients' Needs

The recommendations follow the order in which they are discussed in the text. Priority recommendations are highlighted.

Session cancellations

Recommendation	Action needed by
1 Monitor session cancellation rates and the reasons for them, and put in place systems to reduce their occurrence (for example, by providing incentives for directorates to reduce cancellations and arrange swapping/re-scheduling where cancellation is unavoidable).	**Medical director, clinical directors**

Absence control

2 Issue clearly stated written rules about leave entitlements, when they can be taken, notice required, etc; monitor actual leave taken against the rules.	**Clinical director**
3 Control theatre staff sickness absence.	**Theatre manager**

Matching skills to patients' needs

4 Establish guidelines that differentiate between emergencies (patients who must be operated on immediately); urgent patients who need an operation within four hours; and semi-urgent cases (those who need treatment within 24 hours). By doing this, most operations can be shifted safely to scheduled daytime 'urgent case' sessions. Monitor the number of operations taking place outside scheduled sessions.	**Medical director, clinical directors**

RECOMMENDATIONS

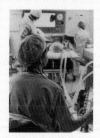

2 Matching Skills to Surgical Patients' Needs

	Recommendation	Action needed by
5	Grade planned operating lists and other kinds of patient activity by complexity, and agree standards about what grade of anaesthetist is appropriate to work, and cover absence, at each level of complexity.	**Clinical director**
6	Sponsor cross-trust research to verify or replace the new system of describing anaesthesia casemix for surgical patients as defined in this report.	**NHS Executive, national professional organisations**
7	Record regularly anaesthesia casemix in relation to the grade of anaesthetist.	**Clinical director**
8	Develop a proactive on-call system, embodied in a written policy, so that subconsultant doctors know when to seek help. Make consultants aware of their specific responsibilities for ensuring that subconsultant doctors do so.	**Clinical director, individual clinicians**
9	Plan to include solo trainee and non-consultant career grade sessions in the rota, matching their skills and experience.	**Clinical director**

Covering for absence

10	Monitor consultants' compliance with their job plan and template rota commitments on a regular basis.	**Medical and clinical director**
11	Designate more of the clinical sessions in consultants' job plans as variable – that is, not fixed in time and place to a particular weekday morning and afternoon – making risk-sensitive cover of absences easier.	**Medical and clinical director**

RECOMMENDATIONS

	Recommendation	Action needed by
12	When consultants' sessions are cancelled (for any reason), they should expect to 'pay back' in the future by covering another consultant's absence when needed.	**Clinical director, individual consultants**

Supervision and training costs

13	Sponsor research to establish whether or not the 'Calman' requirements for shorter training periods can be introduced without incurring extra costs to make good the reduced absence cover provided by trainees.	**NHS Executive**

3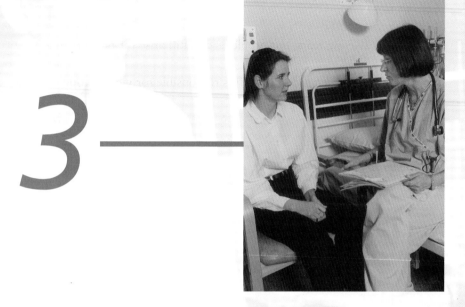

The Quality of Surgical Patients' Anaesthesia Care

Efficient ways of admitting patients – often on the day of surgery, both for day case patients and inpatients – can cause problems for anaesthetists and risk leaving patients anxious and ill informed. Some hospitals are better than others at controlling pain after surgery. Good collaboration between anaesthetists, surgeons and nurses is the key to ensuring that patients are well informed and kept free from pain.

Introduction

86. This chapter looks at the part that anaesthetists play in ensuring that surgical patients are free from anxiety before their operation, and are relieved of pain and anaesthetic side-effects while recovering afterwards. Patients may, of course, have fears about their operation that are of a surgical rather than an anaesthetic nature, but these fall outside the scope of this study and are not considered here. Neither does this chapter consider the individual clinical skill of anaesthetists that goes into making the actual operation a success.[25]

87. Individual anaesthetists may be skilled at interacting with their patients and allaying fears, but problems can still arise for patients that stem from how anaesthetists and other staff interact. Sometimes there is confusion about which group of staff is responsible for what – good co-ordination is needed between the anaesthetist and the surgeon responsible for the patient's overall care, the wider surgical team working in clinics and on the wards, recovery nurses, ward nurses and doctors and nurses specialising in acute pain. Problems may also arise because individual clinicians do not use best practice pain relief methods, and because the mechanisms for helping staff to change their practice are weak.

Information needed before the operation

88. Both the anaesthetist and patient need information before the operation takes place. The anaesthetist needs to decide if the patient is fit for surgery and, if not, what might be done to achieve fitness. Patients need information about what is going to happen to them, to reduce their fears and because they have a right to know. Efficient ways of admitting patients – often on the day of surgery, both for day case patients and inpatients – create time pressures that can cause problems for anaesthetists and risk leaving patients anxious and ill informed.

Patients' worries

89. Patients need an opportunity to discuss the anaesthetist's proposals and, where alternatives are clinically appropriate, to make informed choices between, for example, general or regional anaesthesia, patient- or nurse-controlled analgesia and oral, injection or suppository modes of application. Because unexpected events are more distressing, patients need to know in advance that after surgery they will receive effective and well-co-ordinated pain relief on the ward, and be told about any possible postoperative effects of the anaesthetic (for example, nausea and vomiting). Given the complexity and amount of information that patients are receiving from the anaesthetist, surgeon and ward nurse, verbal information should be backed up by leaflets, and many patients say that they would prefer to see these before they come into hospital.[26]

90. Many patients have concerns about the anaesthetic and how pain will be controlled [**EXHIBIT 22**], but only some get the necessary written information (one-quarter of inpatients across seven trusts, and half of day surgery patients say they received written information about these things before their operation). For example, one hospital has prepared a booklet explaining patient-controlled analgesia (PCA) and how to work the pump, but not all patients report receiving it. Some patients wake up to find themselves unexpectedly attached to a PCA pump.[27] Others wake up with suppositories *in situ*, without having been asked beforehand about their preferred mode of delivery, despite:

- evidence that most patients prefer to take analgesics by mouth and virtually all expect to discuss the option first (for example, Ref. 41);

- no evidence that minor analgesics delivered rectally act better or faster than when swallowed (always providing the patient is able to swallow) (Ref. 42);

- suppositories being more expensive than oral forms of the same drug; and

- a recent well-publicised disciplinary case with serious consequences for the anaesthetist (Ref. 43).

EXHIBIT 22

Patients' worries about their anaesthetic and after-effects before their operation

Many patients have concerns about the anaesthetic and how pain will be controlled.

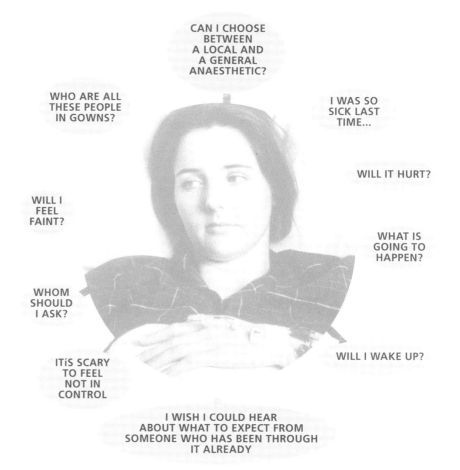

CAN I CHOOSE BETWEEN A LOCAL AND A GENERAL ANAESTHETIC?

WHO ARE ALL THESE PEOPLE IN GOWNS?

I WAS SO SICK LAST TIME...

WILL IT HURT?

WILL I FEEL FAINT?

WHAT IS GOING TO HAPPEN?

WHOM SHOULD I ASK?

ITíS SCARY TO FEEL NOT IN CONTROL

WILL I WAKE UP?

I WISH I COULD HEAR ABOUT WHAT TO EXPECT FROM SOMEONE WHO HAS BEEN THROUGH IT ALREADY

Source: Audit Commission

Effective collaboration is needed to ensure that each patient receives accurate information

91. Sometimes patients do not get the information they need because there is confusion between the surgeon, anaesthetist and nurse about who should inform the patient about pain control. Many patients are unsure who to ask about the different aspects of their hospital stay (for example, about their anaesthetic, pain relief, their condition and what their operation is designed to achieve). Effective collaboration is needed to ensure that each patient receives accurate information, and that patients are not told 'that is not my responsibility, you need to ask X.'

92. Commendably, in Audit Commission surveys only 12 per cent of patients say they spoke to no one before their operation about pain control. Most patients say that they spoke with an anaesthetist before the operation, but fewer patients remember talking with the anaesthetist about how pain would be controlled, despite anaesthetists' expertise in this area. Half of patients remember talking to anaesthetist, surgeon and nurse about pain control, underlining the importance of all three giving consistent advice.

93. The short time available between admission and operation in day surgery units has prompted doctors and nurses to make special efforts to ensure patients are well informed. Guidelines are needed that prompt staff about what to tell patients at each stage, along with rules about recording what they have been told so that omissions can be rectified.

The anaesthetist's visit

94. Although professional standards state that every patient should be visited before their operation, one-third of patients either do not meet the anaesthetist before theatre, or do so for only a few minutes [**EXHIBIT 23A, overleaf**]. This is insufficient time to assess patients fully and answer questions.[28] Difficulties that arise when patients are admitted on the day of surgery can partially be eased by introducing pre-admission clinics [**CASE STUDY 5, overleaf**]. Problems are compounded when anaesthetists cannot find patients quickly [**EXHIBIT 23B, overleaf**] or get little advance warning of whom is on the list. Half of consultants do not receive the names of patients on the list until the day of the operating session, and a further third have only one day's notice.

EXHIBIT 23A

Anaesthetists' contact with patients before their operation

One-third of patients either do not meet the anaesthetist before theatre, or do so for only a few minutes.

EXHIBIT 23B

The main reasons are that many patients are admitted only on the day of surgery, and because anaesthetists cannot find patients quickly.

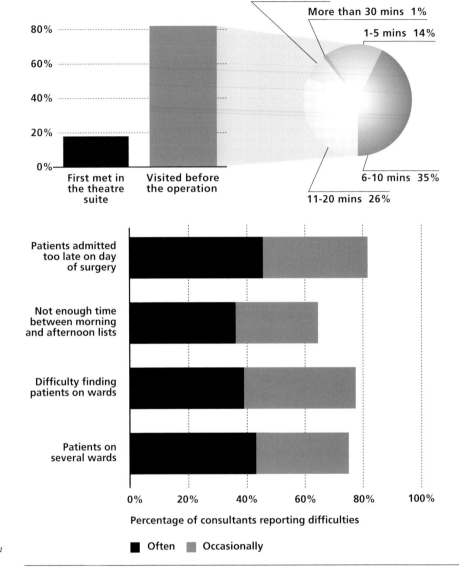

Source: Audit Commission study sites; 539 consultant anaesthetists' questionnaire replies from 45 trusts. Patients' replies from seven trusts report similar visit lengths

CASE STUDY 5

The anaesthetist's visit
Short visits and limited information

A consultant in a large teaching hospital said that most of his lists contained some patients who were late substitutions and who could not be visited beforehand. One particular list is often made up entirely of patients different from those named on the list received the previous day at 4pm. Meeting these patients in the anaesthetic room is sufficient, in his view, to assess whether it is safe to go ahead with the operation, and in reality few operations are cancelled. But he is concerned about patients' anxieties, as anaesthetists do not offer formal training to nurses that helps them to discuss anaesthesia with patients on admission.

CASE STUDY 5 (cont.)

The anaesthetist's visit

Compensating for short visits with generous pre-admission clinic time

At a second trust, patients for a general surgery list are all admitted on the morning of their surgery. The anaesthetist visits them in the hour before his first morning list begins, but is able to spend only a few minutes with each, allowing little time for discussion. However, most patients have attended a pre-admission clinic on the ward, run by a nurse, which covers all aspects of their forthcoming admission. Although nurses have not been specifically trained to talk about the anaesthetic, they can give basic information and discuss pain control.

An 'arrival lounge' in theatre

One hospital receives patients admitted on the day of surgery in a room in the theatre suite, rather than on to wards. This avoids the problem of finding beds on wards in the early morning and allows time for overnight patients to be discharged. It also avoids unnecessary confusion for incoming patients, who do not need a ward bed for the short time before their operation. Nor does the anaesthetist waste time trying to find patients scattered across different wards: time that is then available for talking to the patients.

Generous visit time

At a fourth hospital, the patients for a major orthopaedic list are admitted the day before their operation, and the anaesthetist visits the ward the evening before. The anaesthetist spends about ten minutes with each patient, but more if necessary, giving plenty of opportunity for questions.

Pain after surgery

95. Controlling pain is important for both quality and cost reasons. Effective analgesia may speed or improve recovery and thus shorten lengths of stay [CASE STUDY 6, overleaf] (Refs. 45-50). In only rare cases is pain an indicator of surgical complications[29] – for most patients it is a result of surgery that can be avoided or reduced. Patients' pain remains the overall responsibility of the admitting surgeon, but the anaesthetist also has a separate duty of care to their patients that includes pain relief. To control pain well needs good multidisciplinary teamworking.

CASE STUDY 6

The cost of poor pain control

The financial cost of anaesthesia or analgesia problems is readily demonstrated in day surgery units, because any patient who is too 'sleepy, sore or sick' may have to stay in and occupy an inpatient bed overnight. The patient bears the cost of disruption to arrangements and painful or unpleasant symptoms. There may be opportunity costs for the trust if an inpatient operation has to be cancelled, and extra hotel expenditure and staff costs.

In most trusts only one in twenty, or fewer, patients had to stay in overnight. But in some trusts the stay-in rate is much higher:

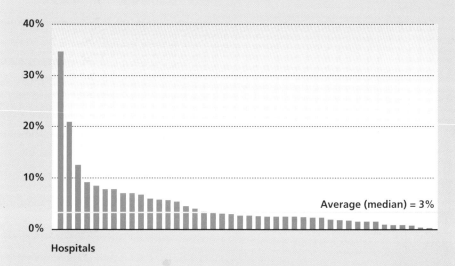

Percentage of day surgery patients actually staying in overnight

Average (median) = 3%

Hospitals

Source: Audit Commission study sites; 42 hospitals in 28 trusts

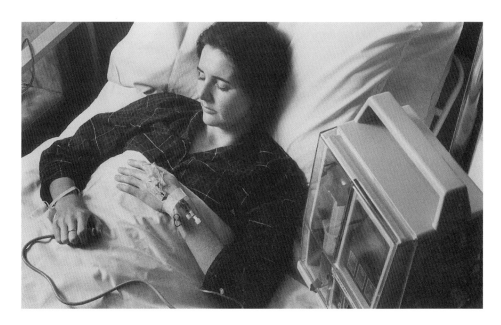

CASE STUDY 6 (cont.)

Reasons for unplanned overnight stays vary widely, but pain and side-effects of anaesthesia are among the most common:

Percentage by reason of day surgery patients staying in overnight

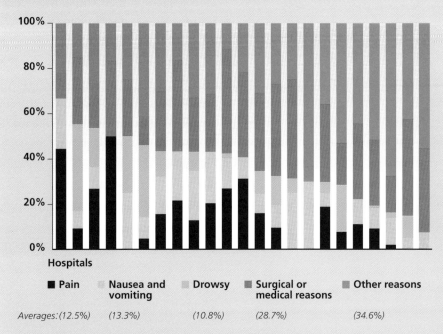

Averages: (12.5%)   (13.3%)   (10.8%)   (28.7%)   (34.6%)

Source: Audit Commission study sites; 23 hospitals in 20 trusts

One day surgery unit audited its stay-in rates after an increase in general surgery necessitated the use of anaesthetists with little previous experience of day surgery. Results for 1,000 cases in 1994 showed that, for all procedures, stay-in rates for the five weekly lists (which had regular pairings of the same surgical team and anaesthetist) varied between 1 and 9 per cent. Anaesthesia and analgesia problems were more often the cause than surgical complications. Forty per cent of one anaesthetist's patients stayed in overnight, compared with rates of between 2 and 10 per cent for the other four lists. The reason identified was a specific problem of analgesic approach: this has since been corrected.

Source: Advisory group member, personal communication

Patients have a right to effective pain relief after surgery, as well as relief from other side-effects such as nausea and vomiting

96. Patients have a right to effective pain relief after surgery, as well as to relief from other side-effects such as nausea and vomiting.[30] A commission of the Royal College of Surgeons and the College of Anaesthetists in 1990 concluded that 'the management of pain after surgery in the UK is unsatisfactory' (Ref. 55). Many staff at hospitals visited during the current study believe that there is scope to improve pain management in their trusts. Many patients still suffer pain, and some hospitals are better at controlling it than others [**EXHIBITS 24A, 24B, 24C**].

97. Pain can be a problem for patients both when they are in hospital and later when they have gone home. Sometimes the reason is inadequate analgesic methods. More often it is because patients 'fall between stools' – the surgeon and anaesthetist at the operation may agree upon a good analgesic prescription, but problems occur later as pain breaks through, or because the patient needs a different drug. There is a confusion of roles between nurses, the trainee surgical team on-call and (if the hospital has one) the specialist pain team. This section looks at these problems, and what can be done about them.

Effective analgesia

98. Postoperative pain has typically been treated either by injection of a fixed dose of opioid every four hours or 'as necessary'. But today, the opportunity for individually tailored pain relief exists, because of:

- the wide variety of available drugs – ranging in strength from opioids, through non-steroidal anti-inflammatory drugs (NSAIDs), to minor analgesics such as paracetamol; and

- the many forms of administration – including, in addition to injection, oral and suppository forms, and continuous or patient-controlled infusion.

99. In the best instances pain control works very well, but the very strength of modern analgesia – the wide range of options available – leads to variation in what is used by anaesthetists, surgeons and wards within the same hospital. In one hospital, the analgesic prescriptions for three patients undergoing the same operation varied, because they were anaesthetised by different people. One was offered patient-controlled analgesia (PCA), two were not. Some had prescriptions written up for the whole of their stay, others only for the day of the operation. Some anaesthetists visited all their patients when back on the wards to discuss pain control, others did not.

EXHIBIT 24A

Patients in pain after surgery

(a) 'Failure to relieve pain is morally and ethically unacceptable' (Royal College of Surgeons and College of Anaesthetists, 1990) – but many patients suffer pain after surgery...

Percentage of patients in pain

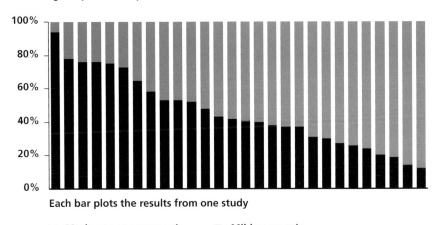

Each bar plots the results from one study

■ Moderate or severe pain   ■ Mild or no pain

EXHIBIT 24B

...and pain continues to be a problem in the 1990s.

Percentage of patients in moderate or severe pain after surgery

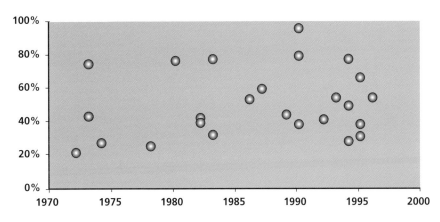

Each point represents the results from one study

EXHIBIT 24C

Some hospitals are better at controlling pain than others, even when casemix is taken into account.

Note: The squares plot the average of all patients' pain for each hospital. The bars show the the variability about the average (+/− standard errors). Hospitals with bars that do not overlap differ significantly in reported pain levels.[31]

Sources: (a and b) published studies and data from Audit Commission site visits;[32] (c) database of 11,053 day surgery patients operated on in 43 hospitals between 1991 and 1995 (only the 19 hospitals with more than 10 hernia patients are plotted)

Pain reported by patients during the 24 hours after their hernia operation

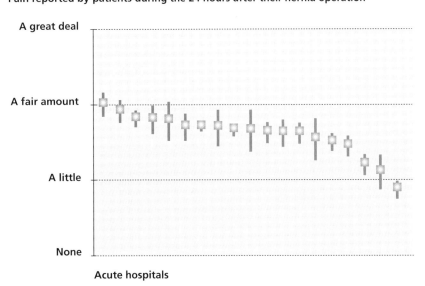

The number of patients using PCA varies between trusts to a degree that is unlikely to be entirely explained by casemix

100. Some hospitals do not have guidelines about when to use the different options; others do, but interviews with patients suggest that they are not always followed. And success becomes critically dependent on ward staff (the trainee surgical team and nurses) having time to monitor patients' pain and the knowledge to make the right decisions about when to change the type or dose of analgesic. This section looks at three options for controlling pain – patient-controlled analgesia, epidurals after major surgery, and minor analgesics in the later postoperative stages.

Patient-controlled analgesia (PCA)

101. PCA pumps allow the patient to self-administer small amounts of analgesic at frequent intervals, rather than receive large doses from a nurse that are hours apart. In theory, PCA provides pain relief that is tailored to an individual patient's needs, and keeps pain at bay all the time. By contrast, injections can result in over-sedation at first, but then allow pain to break through later before the next injection is due. The growth in the use of PCA has been rapid – for example, in one large trust, the number of patients using PCA has grown fourfold in the past three years. The number of patients using PCA varies between trusts to a degree that is unlikely to be entirely explained by casemix (on average, 6 per cent of surgical patients use PCA, with the upper and lower quartiles for 202 trusts being 11 and 4 per cent). A more likely reason for the variation is inequity in the availability of PCA pumps – on average, hospitals have about one available per 1,000 annual patients, but this varies from a lower quartile of one per 500, to one per 1,600.

102. Many published studies have shown that the majority of patients are more satisfied with PCA than with conventional administration of analgesics by a member of staff, although actual pain relief is not necessarily improved (Refs. 57, 58). There is, however, a considerable minority of patients who do not like PCA, either because their pain has not been well controlled by its use, or because of nausea and vomiting (Refs. 59, 60). Patients may experience these problems if they are particularly sensitive to opioids, but also if they have not been prepared in advance (for example, told how to anticipate pain by pressing the button before getting out of bed) or because ward nursing staff have not been trained in how to explain PCA well.[33] Trusts need guidelines to help staff decide who should be offered PCA and, where practicable, use of PCA pumps must be discussed with the patient beforehand.

Epidural analgesia after major surgery

103. Epidural analgesia after major abdominal or thoracic surgery is becoming more common and is reported to offer good pain control. However, unlike PCA, it is more demanding of ward nurses' skills, and requires good training and support to be available. For this reason, although 92 per cent of trusts report using epidurals, 14 per cent state that patients receiving epidural analgesia can be nursed only in ICU, 15 per cent in either ICU or a high dependency unit (HDU), and 30 per cent

To enable more patients to benefit from pain relief, some trusts will need to invest further in the training of ward nurses

in certain designated wards only. In 40 per cent of trusts the same patients may be nursed on any of the surgical wards. To enable more patients to benefit from this form of pain relief, some trusts will need to invest further in the training of ward nurses.

Ineffective drugs in the later stages of pain relief

104. Sometimes pain breaks through if a patient's treatment is changed too quickly from a strong opioid prescription to a minor analgesic. Some of the minor drugs in common use are ineffective: even with the most effective (an NSAID), three in ten patients will not get good pain relief (Ref. 42). With the next most effective drug, only about half will have good relief. And with some of the most commonly prescribed drugs, even fewer patients will have their pain properly relieved. Despite this lack of effectiveness, these drugs are widely used and guidelines based on scientific evidence are rarely available.

105. Break-through pain is especially likely when patients go home. Between 10 and 20 per cent of patients suffer unacceptable levels of pain at home after day surgery (Refs. 61, 62), because they are sent home with, or advised to buy, inadequate minor analgesics. For example, at one hospital, patients were given a letter advising them to buy either of two over-the-counter drugs. They were not told which was likely to be most effective or why, despite the fact that one has been shown to relieve pain in nearly twice as many patients. Other hospitals do better than this [CASE STUDY 7].

CASE STUDY 7

Making sure that pain is controlled after the patient has gone home

One way to improve analgesia advice is to grade operations by likely pain levels. One hospital grades operations as likely to cause mild, moderate or severe pain (for example, cystoscopy, breast surgery and arthroscopic knee surgery, respectively). There are different recommended prescriptions for each, with instructions on what to do at home. The proportion of patients reporting severe pain at home fell once this system had been introduced, as did the number reporting that they were still confined to bed and had disturbed sleep. One reason for the success of this approach might be that the prescriptions were given irrespective of the assessed state of patients' pain on discharge – avoiding both the problems of staff underestimating pain levels and of pain emerging more strongly once the patient was back at home, as is known to occur with some operation types.

While this example relates to day surgery, the principle applies equally to patients discharged after inpatient episodes where the levels of pain can be greater still.

Source: (Ref. 63; see also Ref. 64)

Teamworking and individual patient care

106. Whatever is prescribed, it is crucial that a nurse checks the level of pain experienced by the patient frequently, and alters either the dose or type of drug appropriately. Sometimes analgesia is administered in too light a dose, or too infrequently to be effective. Sometimes this happens because nurses and trainee surgeons feel too busy to monitor pain, or to respond quickly enough to each patient's pain. It can also reflect poor planning and inappropriate views:

- nursing care plans often make inadequate provision for the nursing role in controlling pain [BOX F];

- ward medical and nursing staffs' perceptions of pain levels may differ from those of the patient (for example, Ref. 65);

- some nurses and doctors are reluctant to administer opioids at frequent intervals and over several days because of concerns about side-effects and addiction, although the latter postoperatively is very rare (Ref. 66); and

- patients may fear the needle more than the postoperative pain (or the nurse may think they do), they may not ask for pain relief because they think pain is inevitable, they are afraid of being thought cowardly, or are worried about taking up the nurses' time.

BOX F

The nurse's role in managing pain after surgery

Nurses are the one group of staff who are continually nearby and able to monitor patients' postoperative progress. They are the key to ensuring that patients remain free from pain after the initial prescription by the anaesthetist has worn off; or, if the original plan for analgesia turns out not to be working well, to spotting this failure and seeking advice on a change to the programme. Patients vary considerably in the level of pain that they experience after the same operation and in how effectively different drugs and doses relieve their pain. They also vary in their ways of coping with pain – some benefit most from controlling their own pain via PCA; others want clinical staff to bring pain relief at regular timed intervals; others prefer to keep their drug intake to a minimum (Ref. 100). If nurses can meet these individual needs and stop pain from breaking through, both the patient-nurse relationship and the way that patients view their entire hospital experience will benefit.

One tangible way to support this individual approach to care in a busy ward is to plan well in advance. Each patient's named nurse should produce a written plan, with the involvement of the patient. The plan should document the agreement between nurse and patient for managing pain; it is a crucial aid to continuity of care because when the named nurse is off duty, other nurses will have ready access to what this particular patient needs.

Most surgical wards use pre-printed care plans. If well designed, they can save time and make sure that the basic, common needs of patients are covered. But care plans need space to allow for individualisation; and nurses need to use them properly. None of the plans audited in one hospital showed any individualisation. Pain scores were completed at frequent intervals in recovery, but there was no pain scoring on the wards.

107. Improvements come when pain levels are recorded in the same regular way as other vital signs, and when there are guidelines that require action to be taken when pain levels exceed certain levels.[34] Individual differences between patients mean that while the initial prescription should follow evidence-based guidelines, each patient will need personally tailored care to ensure that they remain pain-free. While the nurse occupies the key place in this jigsaw, success requires all of those involved – surgeons, anaesthetists, nurses and patients – to work together, to communicate well and be clear about their respective responsibilities [BOX G].

BOX G

Managing pain after surgery

Good organisation and teamworking are the keys to ensuring pain-free patients after surgery.

For all patients

- purchasers should include specific standards about pain after surgery in their contracts
- the trust's strategy should describe aims regarding pain control after surgery
- aims need to be translated into policies, standards, and guidelines for clinicians to follow; in-service training about what the trust expects, and audit of achievements are also essential
- resources should be earmarked to match agreed priorities (specialist staff, PCA and other pumps)
- surgeons, anaesthetists, nurses and pain specialists must reach clear agreement about what has been delegated to whom
- consultant surgeons retain overall responsibility for the pain that their patients experience after surgery but anaesthetists also have a separate duty of care

For each individual patient

- make sure that someone is taking care of each step; the patient's named nurse is the most obvious person to check that this is happening.

ADMISSION

- Tell the patient what to expect
- Choice should involve the patient
- Back-up with written information (eg, about PCA)
- Prescribe effectively

KEY STAFF

Admitting nurse
Surgeon and/or anaesthetist

RECOVERY ROOM

- Frequent pain scoring
- Pain controlled before leaving

As appropriate:
- Frequent, small analgesic doses
- Set up PCA

KEY STAFF

Recovery nurse
Anaesthetist

WARD/DAY UNIT

- At least hourly pain scoring
- Listen to what the patient says
- Alter dose/drug vs. pain, nausea and respiratory rate scores

KEY STAFF

Ward/Day nurse
Surgical on-call
Specialist advice

HOME

- Prescribe on basis of expected pain for operation, not on discharge pain score
- Back up with written information
- Liaise with GP, follow up by phone as appropriate

KEY STAFF

Ward/Day nurse
Anaesthetist

Source: Audit Commission, based on recommendations by pain specialists (for example, Refs. 39, 42, 67, 68)

Specific standards on pain relief are rare in the contracts of either health authorities or GP fundholders

A strategic view

108. A strategic view of pain management is needed. But purchasers often remain unaware of the issue, and specific standards on pain relief are rare in the contracts of either health authorities or GP fundholders. Many are surprised when they are told by trusts that some of their patients are in pain and are asked for extra funding for a pain team to reduce the problem. The main purchasing authority makes specific funding provision for only 10 per cent of the acute pain nurse specialists employed by trusts. Despite the fact that more than half of pain nurses are funded internally by money identified at trust board level, many trusts' quality strategies contain no mention of pain, and written standards are rare. That clinicians are keen to improve the provision of pain services is reflected by the fact that funding for one-quarter of specialist pain nurses is found by virement within the anaesthesia directorate budget.[35]

The acute pain team

109. Some trusts have found that with a relatively small investment in an acute pain team,[36] they can make a long-lasting and substantial improvement because the team can:

- offer leadership and form a pool of expert advice;

- make sure that ward staff training takes place;

- provide the impetus for change;

- promote more consistent standards across different wards; and

- act as the focal point for the necessary collaboration between staff.

110. Teams may include anaesthetists and surgeons, pharmacists, physiotherapists and specialist nurses. The doctor in the team often takes the lead in introducing new forms of pain control and guidelines on their use. The team can work with the individual patients who are experiencing the most difficult problems, advise on the most appropriate analgesia and be on-call to advise or assist other staff about difficult cases. In some places, acute pain teams are being replaced by specialist teams that deal with all postoperative side-effects and complications, including pain and symptom control, wound management and tissue viability. The respective responsibilities of team members – and their relationship with the admitting and operating surgeon, anaesthetist and ward nurse – are issues for debate (Ref. 69).

111. In 1997, 57 per cent of UK hospitals have formal acute pain teams, compared with 1990 when only a handful had them; but there is considerable variation between regions of the country [**EXHIBIT 25**]. Two-thirds of trusts with a pain team recognise the contribution of the team's leader in their job plan, most commonly by allocating a consultant anaesthetist to the team for one half-day a week. Trusts with a pain team are more likely to employ a nurse specialist than trusts without a team (89 per cent of trusts as compared with 15 per cent). But not all trusts believe in the concept of the nurse specialist or pain team – for example, one trust without a nurse specialist believes in keeping all nursing responsibility for pain management with the ward nursing team, because it is then clear where the responsibility lies for achieving good standards.

EXHIBIT 25

Acute pain services in UK hospitals

In 1997, 57 per cent of UK hospitals have formal acute pain teams, compared with 1990 when only a handful had them; but there is considerable variation between regions of the country.

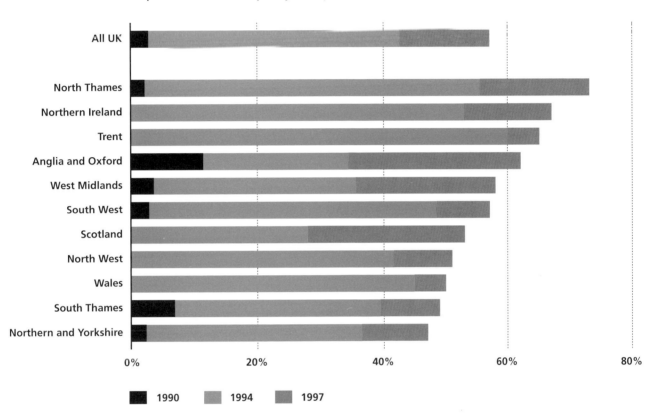

Hospitals with a multidisciplinary acute pain service

Source: 1990 and 1994 figures from Ref. 70 (similar figures for 1994 are reported in Ref. 71); 1997 figures from Audit Commission survey of 304 hospitals across 273 trusts

112. In some hospitals, the introduction of a team with specialist members has been clearly linked to improvements in pain management (Refs. 67, 68, 98). But the existence of a pain team is not enough in itself to ensure successful pain management. The relatively quick turnover of ward nurses and trainee doctors makes the provision of regular in-service training particularly important, because:

- Audit Commission surveys show that even in some hospitals with a pain team, patients are slipping through the net; and

- an audit by anaesthetists at one hospital showed that, although the accuracy of opioid prescribing by trainee doctors improved after guidelines were introduced by the pain team, the majority of prescriptions were nevertheless still incorrect either in dose or frequency (Ref. 72).

Even when a pain team exists, responsibilities must be clarified. Hospitals differ in how the team's role is defined, affecting how many patients' pain is well managed

113. In addition, there are differences in how pain teams operate – of those hospitals with a pain team:

- two-thirds of pain teams undertake regular ward rounds;

- while in 11 per cent of hospitals a team member is present 24 hours a day, seven days a week, in most hospitals the 'general' anaesthetist first on-call attends on request outside normal hours; and

- a team member can be called from home to attend in 19 per cent.[37]

114. In the absence of a pain team some alternative forum for promoting multidisciplinary care is needed – for example, one hospital visited had a pain group that meets regularly and contains an anaesthetist, surgeon, pharmacist, recovery nurses and ward nurses. But even when a pain team exists, responsibilities must be clarified. Hospitals differ in how the team's role is defined, affecting how many patients' pain is well managed. In two-thirds of trusts with a pain team, surgeons have agreed that it should automatically take responsibility for any patient that it thinks needs its service. At the other extreme, in 11 per cent of trusts the pain team does not attend individual patients, restricting its role to that of general advice, training and the development of guidelines. In the remainder of trusts, the pain team is directly involved with individual patients if specifically requested by a surgeon or ward nurse.

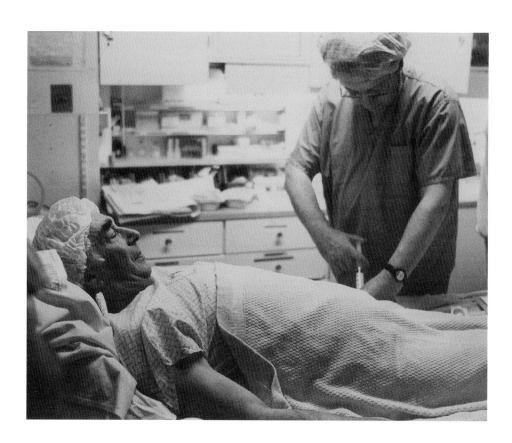

RECOMMENDATIONS

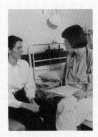

3 The Quality of Surgical Patients' Anaesthesia Care

The recommendations follow the order in which they are discussed in the text. Priority recommendations are highlighted.

Information and anxiety

	Recommendation	Action needed by
1	Agree a policy that states: • who is responsible for giving information about anaesthesia and pain relief to patients – with a multidisciplinary form incorporated in the notes to record who has given information at each stage; • when it is appropriate to offer patients a choice of anaesthetic or approach to pain relief; and • who should be offered patient-controlled analgesia (PCA) – with sufficient equipment/drugs made available to deliver it.	**Chief executive, surgical and anaesthesia clinical directors, director of nursing, individual clinicians**
2	Reinforce verbal information with booklets that explain it in plain language: • what the anaesthetist will do; • what common side-effects and pain patients can expect; • how side-effects and pain will be managed in the hospital and at home afterwards; and • whom to ask if they want more details. Patients should receive written information before they come into hospital for their operation.	**Clinical directors, ward/day unit sisters**
3	Where anaesthetists are unable to visit all patients preoperatively, introduce a systematic way of assigning priorities, to ensure that the most at-risk patients do receive a visit.	**Clinical director**

RECOMMENDATIONS

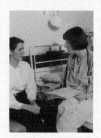

3 The Quality of Surgical Patients' Anaesthesia Care

Recommendation	Action needed by
4 For patients whom the anaesthetist cannot visit, or who are likely to receive only a two-minute visit because they have been admitted on the morning of surgery, train admitting nurses to provide basic information about: • what will happen in the anaesthetic room, during the operation and in recovery; • whom will do what; • who patients will meet; • what types of drug may be used; and • the pain that they are likely to feel, and options for pain control.	**Clinical director**

Pain after surgery

5 Include specific standards about pain relief in contracts; these should include targets – for example, based on the 1992 Welsh Office health gain targets to reduce the percentage of people in severe pain after an operation to under 20 per cent by 1997, and to under 5 per cent by 2002 (Ref. 53).	**Health authorities, GP fundholders**
6 Include a statement of aims towards pain relief in the trust's quality strategy, agreed at board level; these aims should be translated into specific standards, policies and guidelines for staff to follow.	**Director of quality, trust board**
7 Identify one doctor with specialist knowledge of pain relief techniques to promote good practice.	**Chief executive, medical director**

RECOMMENDATIONS

Recommendation		Action needed by
8	Achievements against pain relief targets need regular audit, with patients' pain scores being one of the key quality indicators that are reported regularly to the board.	**Director of quality**
9	Develop evidence-based guidelines on effective analgesic therapies; following these, with frequent pain scoring, is the key to managing pain.	**Clinical director, individual clinicians**
10	Develop a co-ordinated approach to pain management, stemming from a clear agreement on how the anaesthetist will work with the admitting surgeon and other staff to ensure that patients do not suffer unnecessary pain.	**Clinical directors, director of nursing, individual clinicians**
11	The acute pain team should provide written information and guidelines, co-ordinate and educate staff about the management of pain, and provide leadership and a focus for improved teamworking; trusts that do not wish to adopt or fund a formal team approach will need some other mechanism to ensure that these activities take place.	**Chief executive, lead consultant**
12	Develop a programme of continuing education in pain management for trainee doctors and for nurses, because they are in the best position to monitor individual patient progress. The programme should include training on how to incorporate pain relief in the nursing care plan.	**Clinical directors, director of nursing**

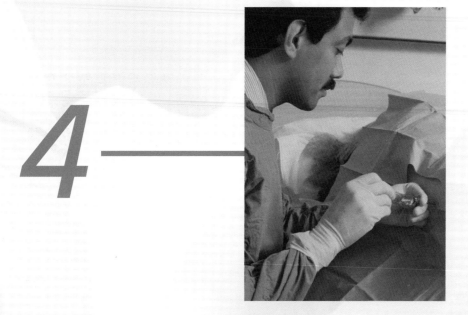

Deciding Priorities Between Surgery and Other Anaesthesia Services

Trusts vary greatly in the resources that they invest in the
non-surgical services, without clear evidence about the
effects on patient care. Better information about workloads
can help trusts to decide on what makes a cost-effective mix
of surgical and other anaesthesia services.
The recommendations call for anaesthetists, the trust board
and purchasers to work together on defining both service
standards for mothers and those in chronic pain, and the
resources needed to deliver them.

Introduction

115. Trusts vary in the number of anaesthetists that they dedicate to different services. On average, three-quarters of clinical sessions are devoted to surgery, but in sampled trusts this proportion varies between two-thirds and four-fifths [**EXHIBIT 26A**]. Some of this variation relates to the size of the trust [**EXHIBIT 26B**], suggesting economies of scale, but this still leaves some similar sized trusts devoting nearly twice as many sessions proportionately to non-surgical services than other trusts.

EXHIBIT 26A

Number of sessions devoted to the different anaesthesia services

On average, three-quarters of clinical sessions are devoted to surgery, but in sampled trusts this varies between two-thirds and four-fifths.*

* 'Other clinical' includes, for example, acute pain, ECT, radiology and 'unallocated' sessions used for absence cover.

Source: Audit Commission, analyses of clinical sessions on template rota from 23 trusts

Percentage of scheduled clinical sessions

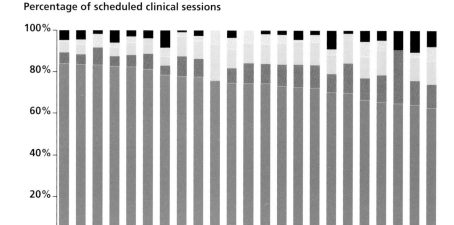

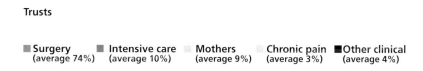

■ **Surgery** (average 74%)   ■ **Intensive care** (average 10%)   ■ **Mothers** (average 9%)   ■ **Chronic pain** (average 3%)   ■ **Other clinical** (average 4%)

EXHIBIT 26B

Some of this variation is related to the size of the trust, suggesting economies of scale.

Source: Audit Commission, analyses of clinical sessions on template rota from 21 trusts

Percentage of anaesthetist sessions in the non-surgical specialties

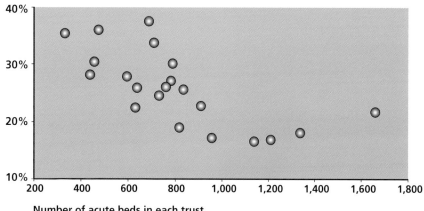

Number of acute beds in each trust

Where there is competition between different clinical services within the same trust for anaesthesia resources, it is up to trust managers and clinicians, in collaboration with their purchasers, to decide on priorities

116. Managers in acute trusts often want to make surgery a priority. Surgery accounts for about half the trust's income. Extra income can be earned through health authority waiting-list initiatives and GP fundholder contracts, which are usually based on cost-and-volume or cost-per-case, and elective surgery can be delayed or reduced to make space for emergency admissions. By contrast, the income from most other areas of service in which anaesthetists work is earned in block contracts – extra activity does not increase income. From anaesthetists' point of view, however, if absence or shortages force them to choose between clinical areas, safety considerations make it more likely that they will cancel elective surgical lists rather than cancel the cover for mothers in emergency or ICU.

117. In some trusts there is a perception that anaesthetists limit the core surgical business by taking on other work. But many anaesthetists believe that the emphasis on their work in operating theatres is misplaced because it misunderstands the range of patients that their skills can help. Anaesthetists have developed treatments in other areas in response to perceived patient need. Where there is competition between different clinical services within the same trust for anaesthesia resources, it is up to trust managers and clinicians, in collaboration with their purchasers, to decide on priorities. The quality of their decisions will be improved if they can make sure that they are investing the right amount of anaesthetist time in each of the different areas. The Audit Commission will report on intensive care services next year. This chapter helps trusts to compare the cost of providing an anaesthesia service in the other two largest areas – maternity and chronic pain – and ensure that care is appropriate and cost-effective.

Mothers

118. Anaesthetists provide key services for mothers during childbirth. As well as caring for emergencies and anaesthetising mothers during caesarean section and other operations, epidural infusion techniques developed by anaesthetists mean that mothers can choose an effective method to relieve normal labour pain. Obstetric anaesthesia presents particular challenges, not least because the 'two lives' involved mean that special care must be taken to ensure that anaesthetic agents do not cross the placental 'barrier' and harm the baby, while at the same time ensuring adequate anaesthesia and pain control for the mother.

119. Trusts must make two basic decisions – first, whether or not the size of the unit, and its distance from the main hospital, justifies continuous resident anaesthetist cover or an on-call service. Units with an anaesthetist in permanent residence are, on average, larger than those that have a resident anaesthetist for part of the time only. But size is only a partial explanation of whether a trust decides to provide permanent cover or not [EXHIBIT 27]. A choice must be made between having anaesthetists dedicated to the service at high cost but minimum risk to mother and baby, and having anaesthetists who are not dedicated to the unit but who are able to respond quickly in an emergency. The distance of the maternity unit from the main hospital is an important factor. Costs are rising as the number of women requiring anaesthesia intervention increases, but also because more trusts are choosing to provide 24-hour resident cover.[38]

120. The second decision is how many consultant sessions to dedicate to the obstetric service. The number of sessions has risen in many trusts over the last decade, and over the same period the number of deaths related to anaesthesia has dropped to low levels (Ref. 73). Anaesthetists involved in obstetrics strongly believe that these two factors are related, as consultant time has been available not only to deliver some of the hands-on care, but also to develop new techniques and monitoring, provide immediate advice, and invest in training and audit. To determine how many consultant sessions are needed, the profession recommends at least one per 500 annual deliveries (Ref. 74). There is no scientific basis for these standards, but they reflect consensus professional judgement, and trusts failing to provide them risk losing College approval. Most trusts under- or over-provide compared with this standard, but there are no comparative data available to say whether there are quality differences that relate systematically to these staffing differences. A considerable number of those over-providing do so because they make sure that there is always a consultant in the unit during normal weekday hours (that is, ten sessions; [EXHIBIT 28]).

121. The potential demand for anaesthetists stems from the number of complex or high-risk cases (for example, mothers who may need resuscitation, or who are at risk of haemorrhage), and is likely to be related to the number of deliveries. But expressed demand is much more immediately linked to the number of caesarean sections and normal labour epidurals for pain control, which together are the reason for four in every five actual anaesthesia interventions. The number of these events varies considerably between trusts – from 10 to 60 per cent of all deliveries [EXHIBIT 29, overleaf].

EXHIBIT 27

Permanent anaesthetist residential cover in relation to the number of mothers delivered

Although there is a significant difference* in size of units between those with and without permanent anaesthetist residence, size only partially explains whether a trust decides to provide permanent cover or not.

Annual deliveries (000)

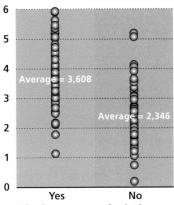

* t=7.55, df=136, p<0.001.

Source: Audit Commission survey of 138 trusts 1996/97

EXHIBIT 28

Consultant anaesthetist sessions in relation to the number of mothers delivered

Most trusts under- or over-provide, compared with the professional standard of at least one weekly consultant anaesthetist session per 500 annual deliveries.

Consultant anaesthetist sessions per week allocated to maternity units

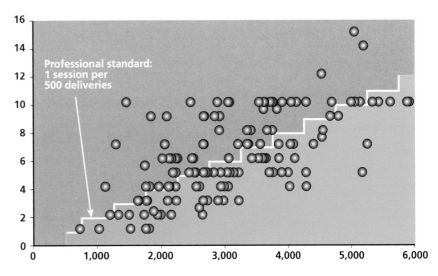

Annual number of women delivered in each trust

Source: Audit Commission survey of 135 trusts 1996/97

EXHIBIT 29

The percentage of women delivered by caesarean section, plus those with an epidural for pain relief during normal labour

The number of caesarean sections and normal labour epidurals for pain control account for four in every five anaesthetist interventions; the rates of such deliveries vary considerably between trusts.

Source: Audit Commission survey of 138 trusts 1996/97

Percentage of caesarean section and normal labour epidurals

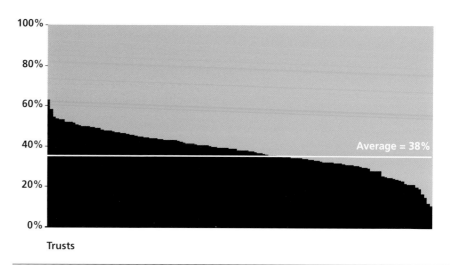

122. Normal labour epidural rates vary most – one trust provided 40 per cent of mothers with a normal labour epidural, while at the other extreme another gave only 5 per cent. The lowest rates might be explained by low anaesthetist staffing levels, but only in some trusts – less than half of the variation in the number of normal labour epidurals is explained by the number of consultant anaesthetist sessions. Some trusts with two consultant sessions give as many epidurals as others with ten sessions. This may mean that trainees are delivering some of these epidurals without receiving an optimal level of training and consultant support. Current consultant staffing levels bear little relationship to the demand for anaesthesia intervention, with trusts of apparently equal workload differing in consultant input by factors of several hundred per cent [EXHIBIT 30].

EXHIBIT 30

Consultant anaesthetist sessions in relation to the number of normal labour epidurals and caesarean section operations

Current staffing levels bear little relationship to the demand for anaesthesia intervention, with trusts of apparently equal workload differing in consultant input by factors of several hundred per cent.

Source: Audit Commission survey of 138 trusts 1996/97

Weekly consultant sessions allocated to maternity units

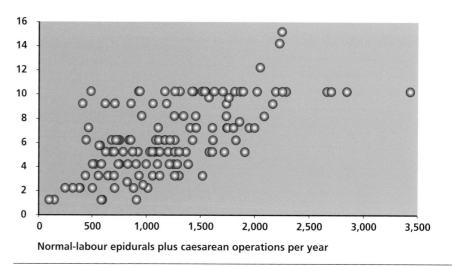

Normal-labour epidurals plus caesarean operations per year

Trusts should decide on the standards that they wish to attain and then determine the staffing levels that are needed to deliver them

123. These findings raise questions for which evidence-based answers are not available. How many anaesthesia events make an appropriate workload for a resident anaesthetist? In some hospitals, resident cover can result in an experienced, expensive anaesthetist being under-employed.[39] On the other hand, not having an anaesthetist present can mean that mothers wait a long time in pain for an epidural, or are not offered a 24-hour epidural service. And what is an appropriate number of consultant sessions? Funding ten normal-hours sessions is expensive but, even so, consultants will miss most of the anaesthesia events, because:

- these are spread across the 24-hour period and at weekends – for example, one hospital found that one-third of events occurred during normal hours, while consultants attended 16 per cent of all interventions; and

- consultants may be called away from the unit. A majority of the consultants surveyed across 42 trusts stated that they spent all of their last obstetric session in the maternity unit, but two out of five were away for spells which lasted from a few minutes to the whole of the session, contrary to professional recommendations (Ref. 74).

124. It might be better to review the number of normal-hours consultant sessions, with a view to providing sufficient cover to ensure good organisation of the service and to promote service developments, new techniques, good training and audit. In some trusts, this review might conclude that it is better to spread out some of the resources to boost staffing levels at other times. Trusts should decide on the standards that they wish to attain – for example, whether a 24-hour epidural service will be offered, the maximum response times to a request, the proportion of elective caesarean operations to be anaesthetised by a consultant, the amount of training and audit effort wanted – and then determine the staffing levels that are needed to deliver them. And because the number of epidurals given is partly influenced by the attitudes of midwives, obstetricians and anaesthetists in addition to the wishes of mothers, it is important that anaesthetists are involved in planning the trust's strategy for childbirth services.

125. Staff availability comes in big step changes (for example, an additional consultant session, or a move from on-call to resident). Trusts risk either stressing staff with too much work, or wasting precious resources. It is not appropriate for the Audit Commission to say what staffing levels should be in relation to workloads, when outcomes have not been measured. Cross-trust research is needed to establish new evidence-based guidelines. In the meantime, trusts can use the method proposed by the Obstetric Anaesthetists' Association, which is based on the number of deliveries, to plan how to cover risk. In addition, they should use the evidence concerning consultant sessions and intervention rates to help them to decide on staffing levels that are also sensitive to actual workloads [EXHIBIT 30, p82]. One trust's experience illustrates how inaccurate staffing levels based on the annual number of deliveries can be.

Had consultant sessions been set according to the number of deliveries, one consultant session should have been dropped in 1995 because there were 500 fewer deliveries than in the previous year; but in fact both the caesarean section and normal labour epidural rate increased, so that in reality there was 10 per cent more work to do. Geographical layout, the need to provide adequate training and the experience of anaesthetists below consultant level who staff the unit, also need to be taken into account.

People with long-lasting pain

Anaesthetists have specialist knowledge about the ways in which the body and brain register pain and how drugs can reduce some types of pain

126. Short-term pain follows most surgery and may also serve as a warning that something is wrong with our bodies. But long-lasting pain is often characterised as 'useless', bringing misery, loss of income and self-respect, and damaging family relationships and friendships (for example, Ref. 75). Intractable pain can vary from continuous but non-life-threatening conditions such as back pain and arthritis, through to the most debilitating pain associated with terminal conditions. It affects very large numbers of people.[40] For example, back pain is the main reason for 20 per cent of all visits to a GP, with the annual cost of NHS treatment nearly £500 million, plus half as much again for non-NHS treatment, plus over £5 billion in terms of lost working time and social security benefits (Ref. 78). Little is known about how many people need a service beyond that of a GP.

Pain clinics

127. By definition intractable pain is difficult to treat, and doctors and therapists from different backgrounds are involved in diagnosing and managing the many different kinds and causes of pain. Some patients progress through the healthcare system by referral between different specialists in a clinically appropriate and efficient way. But others endure a long search – often over many years – around different parts of the NHS and private sector seeking respite prior to their arrival in a chronic pain clinic. Patients referred to one clinic with back pain had been suffering for an average of nine years; patients with different kinds of neuralgia pain for between three and nine years; and those with amputation pain for an average of thirteen years (Ref. 79).

128. Since anaesthetists have specialist knowledge about the ways in which the body and brain register pain and how drugs can reduce some types of pain, they should be one of the key disciplines involved in providing services. Ideally pain clinics staffed by multidisciplinary teams would take appropriate referrals direct from GPs, and plan a package of care that is suited to each person. But in the UK there are few fully multidisciplinary clinics. Partially multidisciplinary clinics led by anaesthetists are the most common type of provision, but nearly one-third are anaesthetist-only clinics [TABLE 3].[41]

TABLE 3

Variations in staffing of chronic pain clinics

Fully multidisciplinary	Clinics staffed by anaesthetists and doctors from several other specialties, plus other specialist staff (for example, nurse, psychologist, physiotherapist, pharmacist)	Uncommon
Partial multidisciplinary	Anaesthetist-led with a doctor from at least one specialty, plus other staff	About one in every five clinics
	Anaesthetist-led with at least one other non-medical specialist member of staff (nurse or therapist)	About two in every five clinics
Single discipline	Anaesthetist-only service	About one-third of clinics

Source: Audit Commission, study site data from 27 trusts (4 further trusts that replied provide no service)

Levels of investment in services for patients with long-lasting pain are variable

129. Levels of investment in services for patients with long-lasting pain are variable, with some populations having no local access at all, and with doctors in some pain clinics seeing twice as many patients per session as in others. A professional standard is to provide ten consultant sessions per 200,000 population (Ref. 39), but as with the obstetric standard referred to earlier, this standard is based on professional judgement and not research evidence. This level of service is rarely if ever attained, and to reach it nation-wide would require a very large increase in the number of consultant anaesthetists within the NHS. In fact the largest service has 23 doctor sessions and provides for over 7,000 attendances and treatments a year. But the most common provision is three to four consultant anaesthetist sessions a week.

Efficient clinics that offer effective treatments can cover their own costs within the trust and provide relief for a needy and neglected group of patients

130. In many trusts contract income does not cover the cost of even these limited services, partly because the anaesthetists in charge are rarely involved in contract discussions with health authorities and GP fundholders. In one trust, outpatient activity was twice – and inpatient activity four times – the levels funded through contracts. The pressure of demand is such that even with extra sessions over contract, only a minority of sites meet the Patient's Charter standard of a 13-week maximum wait for a first outpatient appointment.

131. If activity exceeds contract income, other services are in effect subsidising the chronic pain clinic. Health authorities need to consider the type and levels of service that they wish to fund, and not simply pay for services that are being developed 'ad hoc' by clinicians that reflect their individual interests and experience. Efficient clinics that offer effective treatments can cover their own costs within the trust and provide relief for a needy and neglected group of patients.

Effective treatments

132. Most clinics provide a range of treatments. But those patients with the most intractable pain may not be cured or even have their pain relieved as a result of their treatment.[42] At one trust, doctors hoped that they made people's lives easier, but were under no illusions – they had no data about outcomes, and mostly offered a consulting diagnostic service. A recent critical evaluation for the Health Technology Assessment programme found that many of the treatments offered at pain clinics in the UK are effective, but there is insufficient evidence to know whether the remainder can be recommended for continued use (Ref. 84). Examples of treatments about which trusts need to think carefully – because their effectiveness has not been scientifically proved – are transcutaneous nerve stimulation (TENS), acupuncture and spinal cord stimulators.

133. Despite this lack of evidence, many clinics are providing some procedures that involve medium to high cost and risk which have been shown by science to be without effect (Appendix 6). By contrast, fewer clinics offer a psychological service, although there is evidence that this can improve quality of life (Ref. 84).[43] Purchasers and trusts should compare the treatments offered locally with the framework described in Appendix 6 as an aid to designing an appropriate portfolio of services. Pain clinics specialising in a particular type of treatment may not match this framework, in which case purchasers should also have contracts with a nearby generalist clinic.

Pain clinicians do not know whether a low or high number of repeat attendances means better outcomes: more comparative audit is needed

Efficient clinics

134. Pain clinics can increase the number of patients that they treat for a given level of resources by reviewing follow-up attendances. The average number of attendances per outpatient in this study varied from 1.5 to 9.5, with most trusts in the range 2.0 to 3.5. These variations are not readily explained by casemix – for example, a study of ten clinics found that in one clinic 43 per cent of patients with lower back pain were seen more than once, as compared with 79 per cent in another, and that the more time that clinicians spent seeing repeat patients, the longer the waiting times for new patients to be seen (Refs. 86, 87). Some clinics have agreed referral guidelines with local GPs, and a policy for when discharge from the clinic is appropriate. Pain clinicians do not know whether a low or high number of repeat attendances means better outcomes: more comparative audit is needed to identify optimum attendance frequencies – that is, those that provide patients with what they need without incurring unnecessary cost and lengthening waiting times for others.

135. Expensive staff – for example, consultant anaesthetists – should not spend time delivering treatments that others could provide as effectively at lower cost. Some trusts add nurses and therapists to the team [**BOX H**]. One trust calls the nursing sisters 'case managers': they not only spend more time with patients than do consultants, but provide continuity during the course of a treatment package, helping to ensure that the patient is supported through it without needing to see the consultant on each follow-up visit.

BOX H

Ensuring that chronic pain clinics run efficiently

There is some scope in clinics to use nurses or therapists to carry out some of the work that doctors do – for example, acupuncture and TENS – that can improve the cost efficiency of the clinic. For example:

- the consultant prioritises referrals according to the urgency of the patient's condition and severity of pain;

- the specialist nurse sees selected patients in a nurse-led clinic for preliminary assessment and start of treatment, if this is appropriate. This approach can save the patient a long wait to see the consultant which may, in any case, be unnecessary;

- the consultants have a discharge policy;

- telephone follow-up should be used where appropriate instead of automatically booking a return appointment;

- the specialist nurse, physiotherapist and occupational therapist provide a range of complementary treatments; and

- open access clinics are provided for patients to see the specialist nurse.

Cost effectiveness

136. It has been proposed that, far from being an extra cost, pain clinics could pay for themselves by reducing the consumption of other NHS resources.[44] Evidence from the UK is lacking, apart from one study showing reduced drug costs (£240 per patient reduction a year) and describing an unquantified reduction in hospital treatment costs (Ref. 89). Because of this lack of evidence, the Audit Commission asked one pain clinic to carry out a small study which showed that the clinic covered its cost by reducing consumption elsewhere within the acute trust. There were also cost savings to the NHS in terms of significantly reduced GP consultations and to the patients themselves, by significantly reducing their private treatment costs (Appendix 6).

137. National research is needed to provide this type of information, so that trusts and purchasers can design local services to improve quality of life while reducing costs elsewhere in the system. The same need for national research has been identified with regard to maternity services – at the moment trusts and purchasers do not have good information to help them to determine appropriate staffing levels and priorities between different services. These changes cannot be achieved by individual clinicians alone, but require management action. This is a common theme of many of the findings of the first four chapters, and is the subject of the next chapter.

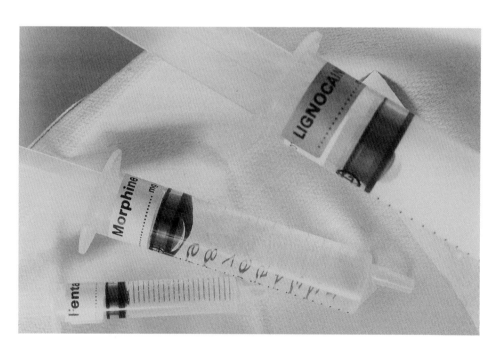

RECOMMENDATIONS

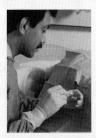

4 — Deciding Priorities Between Surgery and Other Anaesthesia Services

The recommendations follow the order in which they are discussed in the text. Priority recommendations are highlighted.

Mothers

	Recommendation	Action needed by
1	Sponsor research to establish new evidence-based guidelines for determining staffing levels and grade mix for obstetric anaesthesia so that the national standard relating anaesthesia input to delivery rates can be revised to take account of anaesthesia event-rates.	**Royal College of Anaesthetists, Obstetric Anaesthetists Association, NHS Executive**
2	Review anaesthetist staffing provision in the light of the caesarean rate and normal labour epidural rate, and not solely on the number of deliveries. Monitor annual changes in anaesthesia event-rates.	**Chief executive, clinical director, lead consultant for obstetric anaesthesia**
3	Involve anaesthetists in planning the trust's strategy for childbirth services, because the normal labour epidural rate is partly influenced by the attitudes of anaesthetists, as well as those of midwives, obstetricians and mothers.	**Chief executive, clinical directors for obstetrics and anaesthesia, director of midwifery, lead anaesthetist**

Chronic pain

	Recommendation	Action needed by
4	Estimate the need for chronic pain services.	**Health authorities, GP fundholders**
	Sponsor research to guide local purchasing authorities in estimating the need for chronic pain services, taking into account the wider cost-benefit trade-offs between investment in the pain clinic, and reduced expenditure in other areas (for example, GP consultations, consultations with and procedures given by other NHS specialties).	**NHS Executive, national professional organisations**

RECOMMENDATIONS

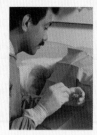

4 Deciding Priorities Between Surgery and Other Anaesthesia Services

	Recommendation	Action needed by
5	Review chronic pain treatments on offer in the light of the evidence of their effectiveness; in line with NHS Executive recommendations, purchasers should reduce funding for treatments that good evidence has shown to be without effect and increase expenditure on those shown to be effective.	**Health authorities and GP fundholders, lead clinician**
6	Include outcome standards relevant to a chronic pain service in purchasing contracts (that is, about psychological support, quality of life, rehabilitation, improved functioning). Such standards should be similar to those for other chronic illnesses (for example, asthma or chronic bronchitis), and should consider the inter-agency co-ordination required.	**Health authorities and GP fundholders**
7	Draw up a business plan that includes an assessment of the demand for the chronic pain service, and which identifies the particular services, the range of treatments and staffing to be provided.	**Lead clinician, directorate manager**
8	Involve the lead chronic pain clinician in contract discussions to ensure that a realistic contract is signed; then monitor expenditure and activity against contract values.	**Chief executive, lead clinician, directorate manager**
9	Review the number of follow-up outpatient appointments per chronic pain patient to ensure that they are clinically appropriate. Agree referral guidelines with GPs, and a discharge policy.	**Lead clinician, individual clinicians**
10	Ensure that expensive doctor time is not spent delivering treatments (for example, acupuncture) that cheaper staff can provide as effectively.	**Clinical director, individual clinicians**

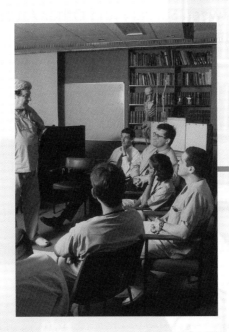

5

Leadership and Change

This report sets out a challenging agenda for change. The hallmarks of a value-for-money directorate are listed and can be used for self-audit. But in many cases too little time is given to clinical directors, and for others frustration develops because they lack the power to make changes. Some of the changes need wider debate, either because they go beyond the specialty of anaesthesia, or look ahead to the next millennium.

Introduction

In many trusts clinical directors have neither the time, training nor the power to achieve all the changes required

138. The great majority of changes recommended in earlier chapters need action at directorate level. Trusts must manage these changes well to protect the two-thirds of income that is underpinned by anaesthetists. But in many trusts clinical directors have neither the time, training nor the power to achieve all the changes required. This problem is not unique to anaesthesia directorates, and poses wider questions for the NHS as a whole.

139. Previous chapters have identified the attributes that distinguish directorates that deliver good value for money. Directorates can use a summary of these attributes as a basis for self-audit [BOX I]. The rest of this chapter considers:

- organisational development (the effects of different directorate structures on the management of anaesthesia resources; the role of the clinical director; the balance required between individual consultant freedoms and the corporate needs of the trust);

- key quality and cost improvements; and

- future challenges (whether the deployment of non-medically trained staff – used elsewhere in the developed world – might reduce the future demand for doctors in the UK; and the changes needed to medical staff planning).

BOX I

The 50 hallmarks of a value-for-money anaesthesia directorate

What does a high quality anaesthesia directorate look like? One that has few of the problems outlined in the preceding chapters, obviously. Anaesthesia directorates can use this Audit Commission summary as a checklist for self-audit:

Ensures good quality

- provides a high standard of anaesthesia and analgesia;

- sets clear standards and values that take into account guidelines issued by the Royal College of Anaesthetists, Association of Anaesthetists, General Medical Council and other relevant bodies;

- develops evidence-based guidelines, audits achievement, and acts to ensure compliance with guidelines;

- has good written information for patients about the different types of anaesthetic (general, local, regional), pain and the side-effects that can be expected and what will be done to alleviate them;

- makes sure that every patient receives the right written information, either by providing it directly or ensuring that the admitting nurse does so;

BOX I (cont.)

- develops a system to ensure that priority patients receive a visit by the anaesthetist of adequate length;

- ensures that ward or day unit nurses have been trained to discuss the basics of the anaesthetic and pain-relief techniques likely to be used, especially when admitting regimens restrict the time that anaesthetists can spare to talk to patients; and

- ensures that subconsultant doctors do not anaesthetise complex patients.

Plans ahead

- has an up-to-date business plan with time-limited objectives that are assigned to specific individuals;

- plans costed responses to developments in surgical and other directorates' plans;

- plans how to meet future costs – for example, assesses whether New Deal costs could be met by reducing costs due to session cancellations;

- plans response to expected changes in patient numbers in each care group;

- considers how the trust can meet the demands of the New Deal and Calman; and

- calculates the trade-off between investment in different services when anaesthetists are in short supply.

Communicates effectively with its own and other staff

- communicates effectively with its staff;

- links with other directorates (for example, sends lead consultants to other directorates' meetings);

- has a forum for encouraging and discussing feedback from those directorates that see themselves as 'users' of the anaesthesia directorate's services;

- has good ongoing communications with surgical secretaries about list changes and planned absences, allowing for re-scheduling and reduction of cancellations;

- informs anaesthetists if their expenditure on agents and drugs is different from the average;

- has written agreement with surgeons about their responsibilities for monitoring and relieving pain throughout the patient's stay and at home afterwards; and

- trains nurses and trainee surgeons in pain relief.

cont./

BOX I (cont.)

Matches staff resources to contracts

- helps the trust to employ the range of skills needed to deliver anaesthesia and pain relief services throughout the hospital;

- analyses the anaesthesia event-rate in maternity and provides an appropriate number of consultant sessions;

- agrees contracts for chronic pain that match resources input; and

- monitors activity against contracts.

Is a good employer

- appraises consultants and other staff, linking personal development needs to those of the directorate and the trust;

- involves trainee and non-consultant career grades in audit;

- creates a culture that allows part-time working and other good recruitment and retention techniques;

- has tried other options for reducing shortages – for example, linked posts with universities, paying for extra sessions;

- offers high-quality training;

- keeps actual trainee doctor hours to New Deal requirements;

- offers non-consultant career grades continuing education opportunities, and monitors the quality of their work;

- works with the medical director to develop a set of job plans with as close to seven clinical commitments per anaesthetist as possible;

- designs a template that translates contracted commitments into an efficient rota that provides sufficient solo and directly supervised lists for trainees;

- devises on-call systems of reasonable frequency and intensity;

- controls incremental drift;

- has optimal ODA/anaesthetic nurse grade mix and staffing levels;

- looks to minimise expensive temporary staff costs (locums, agency);

- has a policy on ODA enhanced roles, and has explicit reasons for extending roles; and

- has progressed on ODA/theatre nurse multi-skilling.

Covers absences

- keeps session cancellations to the bare minimum;

- meets standards for advance notice about absences, allowing sessions to be re-scheduled;

- contracts some anaesthetists to provide unallocated sessions, to cover for absences; and

- ensures that session complexity matches the skill of the cover anaesthetist.

BOX I (cont.)

Develops a sound physical environment

- provides modern equipment in each theatre that ensures safety without excessive duplication or downtime in usage;

- has procurement and maintenance plans that reduce costs via tendering and single-supplier volume-purchase discounts;

- has a formulary which includes expensive alternatives only when clinically indicated, and monitors usage against guidelines; and

- invests in low-flow equipment and ensures payback by training staff and monitoring the achievement of low flows.

Structure encourages value for money

- has a properly resourced business manager and administrative staff;

- gives those with most influence over expenditure responsibility for budgets;

- identifies a lead for each main clinical area; and

- provides a reasonable number of sessions for management tasks.

Organisational development

Structures

140. In the great majority of trusts the clinical directorate is the structure through which the changes that this report recommends will be implemented. All trusts group anaesthetists together as a separate department, and there are no examples in the UK where anaesthetists are split up and placed managerially within the directorates for which they provide a service. This structural arrangement makes it easier for anaesthetists to provide flexible cover and to deal with training and other professional activities. To prevent isolation, good communication with other specialties is therefore crucial – for example, about theatre list content and changes, and the assignment of responsibilities and the teamworking needed to manage pain after surgery. Some trusts try to foster good communication by placing anaesthetists as a group within a larger surgical directorate that may be led by either an anaesthetist or a surgeon, with the different surgical specialties and anaesthesia heads forming a directorate board. In others, anaesthesia stands alone. Whatever the wider directorate structure, the anaesthesia department's budgets should include all expenditure that is within anaesthetists' control, including the cost of drugs and consumables used in theatres. This does not always happen [TABLE 4, overleaf].

TABLE 4

How management responsibilities for anaesthesia-related services are aligned in different trusts

Location within the trust	Trusts						
	A	B	C	D	E	F	G
Separate directorate	✓	✓		✓	✓	✓	
Sub-directorate of surgical directorate			✓				✓
Managed by anaesthetists?							
Staff							
ODAs	✓	✓	✓	✓	✓?	✗	✗
Theatre staff	✓	✓	✓	some	✗	✗	✗
Recovery staff	✓	✓	✓	some	?	✗	✗
Equipment and drugs							
Anaesthetic equipment budget (capital)	?	some	some	some?	?	✗	✗
Maintenance budget	✓?	✓?	✓?	some	?	some	✗
Anaesthetic consumables budget	✓?	✓	✗	some	?	✗	✗
Anaesthetic drugs budget	✓?	✓	✗	some	?	some	✗
Units							
Day surgery unit	✓	✓	✓	✗	✗	✗	✗
Operating theatres	✓	✓	✓	some	✗	✗	✗
Intensive care units	✓	✓?	✓	✓	✓	✗	✗
Acute pain management teams	✓	✓	✓	✓	n/a	✓	n/a
Chronic pain service	✓	✓	n/a	✓	✓	n/a	✓

Source: Audit Commission site visits (n/a = no service; ? = unclear or not known)

The clinical director as a focus for change

141. Most anaesthesia directorates have:

- a consultant as director;

- lead anaesthetists for each of the main service areas; and

- a general manager, to whom a theatres manager, ICU senior nurse and a senior ODA may report.

EXHIBIT 31

Anaesthesia clinical directors' clinical commitments

Some clinical directors may lack time for management, because they drop only one clinical session, and some do not drop any.

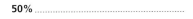

Percentage of trusts

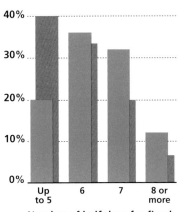

Number of half days for fixed clinical commitments

Smaller trusts (between 300 and 800 beds)

Larger trusts (between 825 and 1,725 beds)

Source: Audit Commission, analyses of job plans from 40 trusts

142. Some anaesthesia departments display more of the characteristics set out in Box I than others, but few – perhaps none – would claim to be entirely successful. The blame does not rest solely with the doctors. Purchasers and trust boards have a responsibility for creating the conditions in which this kind of directorate-based self-governance can develop and prosper (Ref. 91). One of the major difficulties is that, while some clinical directors take a keen interest in management, others see it as a distraction from clinical duties; an onerous, often thankless task at which individual consultants are obliged to take turns. Some clinical directors may be able to find the time for their management duties by changing how they spend their flexible commitment time. But those who drop only one clinical session, or none, may not have enough time for management [EXHIBIT 31].[45] Clinical directors can agree to work fewer clinical sessions, but frequently choose not to reduce their clinical commitments but to be paid instead for additional work. Most clinical directors retain five or six clinical sessions, while one-third work seven or more clinical sessions and add their directorate duties on top.

Individuals and the whole

143. In addition to structure and time constraints, the other key barrier to clinical directors' effectiveness is their formal relationship with their consultant colleagues. Clinical directors do not have direct management responsibility for consultants; traditionally, doctors work to peer review rather than managerially imposed targets. This approach to working is not unique to anaesthesia, or to medicine – indeed, it is a hallmark of many professions. But a great many of the problems identified in this report cannot be solved unless individual anaesthetists, and the staff working with them, change the way that they do things.

144. There are two aspects to the changes required. First, in order to meet the needs of the service, consultants need to identify with the services provided by the hospital as a whole. Most anaesthetists have a strong sense of commitment to the specialty – membership of professional bodies is high, and many take part in specialty interest groups and meetings across different trusts – but they do not necessarily identify with the trust. And yet their behaviour as individuals has much wider consequences for the whole. The cost and quality consequences of how flexible anaesthetists are at covering absences is a good example of this (Chapter 2).

145. Second, what is the right balance between individual clinical freedom – the principle of doctors applying their own judgement to the care of individual patients – and the limits that should be put on it if it is producing less than the best possible care? Many directorates have some clinical guidelines, but they rarely audit compliance with them and, when they do, there are no mechanisms for ensuring compliance unless serious misconduct has occurred. But this report has shown that inconsistent practice is leaving some patients ill informed and in unnecessary pain. What should be done to ensure that practice is based on evidence and that good practice (where it has been identified) is adopted?

The reasons why the numbers of sessions delivered differ are complex and vary between trusts

146. Clinical directorates need leadership and clinical directors should be well placed to work with their consultant colleagues to set individual objectives that are clearly related to the needs of patients, the directorate and the trust. They need to be able to develop a sense of shared responsibility while devolving decision-making and accountability, and to foster strong motivation and morale among staff. Performance review is one way of ensuring good use of resources and quality of work by those with devolved responsibilities, and the achievement of corporate objectives. Fairly common among directorate management and secretarial staff, it remains rare among doctors.

147. The Association of Anaesthetists and Royal College of Anaesthetists have established a joint working party on good practice in anaesthesia. One of its aims is to help to bridge the gap between the responsibilities of individual doctors for their own self-assessment and professional development, and that of national bodies for issuing standards for the profession as a whole. It aims to help local directorates to develop and adopt standards that can be agreed as corporate benchmarks to which all involved are committed. Programmes such as Oxford and Anglia's 'Getting research into practice' aim to improve individual performance; accreditation of doctors through formal continuing professional development may also develop (Refs. 90, 91, 93).

148. At the moment, clinical directors do not have the authority to bring about the kinds of change that are needed. The debate about the limits to clinical freedom and the sanctions required when the quality of care falls short goes well beyond this specialty and the remit of this report. The issues are beginning to be raised, but the challenge of culture change remains daunting.

The key quality and cost challenges

149. Earlier chapters have touched on the importance of good collaboration and communication between clinicians from different specialties, and clear agreement about areas of responsibility. In particular, the anaesthesia directorate interacts closely with surgery, obstetrics and those involved in palliative care and chronic pain. Within those directorates, there is close contact between anaesthetists and admitting consultants, the trainee surgical teams and ward nurses. Daily working contact makes good partnerships and a team approach between individuals essential. At directorate level more formal mechanisms – such as regular joint meetings – are needed. With effective communication and collaboration, patients are more likely to feel well informed, involved in decisions and free from avoidable pain.

150. Tackling high and rising costs will not be easy. Much of the difference in the cost per session of anaesthetists' clinical work is explained by differences in the number of sessions delivered per anaesthetist.[46] But the reasons why the numbers of sessions delivered differ are complex and vary between trusts. In one trust, the main reason may be how absence is covered, in another it may be supervision levels, or the number of commitments in job plans. No single explanation is common to all trusts.

TABLE 5

The scale of cost variations between trusts by reason

Reason	Annual cost difference*	Basis for comparison
Doctors		
Low service contribution by trainees (that is, few clinical sessions carried out solo; most sessions are worked 'doubled up' with a consultant)	£160,000	UQ** vs. LQ; an UQ trust providing a high level of directly supervised sessions spends at least £160,000 more to deliver the same clinical workload as an LQ trust
High level of direct supervision of non-consultant career grade doctors by consultants	£68,000	UQ vs. LQ
Rich anaesthetist grade mix	£125,000	UQ vs. LQ
High number of consultant absences covered by a non-consultant career grade doctor, trainee or locum rather than by another consultant	£40,000	UQ vs. LQ
In rare cases: five rather than seven half-days for fixed commitments per consultant	Up to £250,000	Most trusts already contract for seven; high extra costs might apply in a few trusts if all consultants are contracted for five rather than seven, and there are no extra workload factors to explain the difference
Theatre staff		
Rich theatre staff grade mix	£140,000	UQ vs. LQ

* Values given are for an average-sized trust.

** UQ (upper quartile) means the most costly 25 per cent of trusts, LQ (lower quartile) the least costly 25 per cent; the values cited are the difference between the trusts occupying the 25th and 75th percentiles, and are thus more conservative than the difference between the true extremes.

Source: Audit Commission study sites

151. However, it is possible to give broad estimates of the relative importance of the various cost drivers across the randomly-selected sample of trusts involved in this study [TABLE 5]. The methodology is not refined and the calculations are rough, but the biggest individual cost components relating to anaesthetist staffing are:

- levels of supervision;
- grade mix; and
- the number of consultant absences covered by trainees, non-consultant career grades or locums rather than by other consultants.

152. For example, differences in the grade mix of consultants, other career grades and trainees mean that trusts in the upper quartile pay anaesthetists an average of at least £52,000 per whole-time equivalent, compared with £47,000 or less in the lower quartile. For an average-sized trust employing 25 anaesthetists, the annual cost difference between the two quartiles is £125,000. A further big cost contributor is differences in theatre staff grade mix.

Future challenges

153. This report has described ways to offset the cost of rising demand by efficiency improvements and to improve quality within the present framework. But in the future it is uncertain whether these measures will be enough to meet the challenges set by reducing trainee service contributions. One radical way forward is to reconsider the issue of non-physician anaesthetists. Another is to re-examine the nature of the consultant's contract.

Non-physician anaesthetists

More radical solutions may be needed to cope with expanding demands in the next century

154. The most serious challenge for the future is the increasing number of patients who need treatment, and the diminishing availability of trainee doctors to carry the burden of front-line treatment. Doctors are increasingly airing these issues in the medical press. Previous chapters have shown how trusts can reduce costs and improve quality within the current framework. Extended role developments seen so far in the UK, described in Chapter 1, do not reduce the demand for doctors, nor do they give consultants more time for training, audit, research, management, overseeing patients with advanced forms of pain management or other activities. More radical solutions may be needed to cope with expanding demands in the next century.

155. The most fundamental way to reduce demands for more doctors substantially would be to adopt the anaesthesia system used in many other countries in the world, including much of Europe and the United States – that is, allowing non-medically qualified staff to maintain anaesthesia under the indirect supervision of doctors who move between two or more operating theatres. Such mid-level practitioners are frequently called 'nurse anaesthetists', although they do not have to come from a nursing background. The extent to which this system can solve problems depends on how it is organised – for example, how many theatres one doctor covers, the training, pay levels and available supply of the non-medically trained staff, and whether they work alone or themselves have support staff.[47]

156. Many UK anaesthetists are concerned about the safety of the non-medically trained staff used in other countries, although others suggest that advances in monitoring equipment make it safer for doctors to be absent from the operating theatre. There have been no comparative international studies that successfully separate the effect of the type of staff administering anaesthesia from all other possible causes of mortality.[48]

157. The Association of Anaesthetists is opposed to the concept of allowing others to induce or maintain anaesthesia without a medically qualified anaesthetist present (Ref. 17), and a recent NHS Executive document did not recommend the introduction of any such scheme (Ref. 96). But the Audit Commission shares the view of some anaesthetists interviewed, that the UK should conduct carefully controlled research, via pilot schemes, to evaluate the boundaries between different staff groups, the financial and patient care implications of change, and the potential for freeing consultants from tasks that might not make the best use of their skills and time.

158. But the development proposed here could bring such benefits. It might begin with a trial involving operating sessions that require two anaesthetists. These are often staffed by a pairing of a consultant and a trainee. As the availability of trainees lessens, a trial involving non-medically trained staff to replace the trainee could be an option. If successful, trials involving a consultant supervising non-medically trained staff in two operating theatres might be tried.

159. Until research takes place, these key questions remain unanswered:

- To what extent could developments solve difficulties in recruiting consultant anaesthetists or in replacing the diminishing service contribution of trainee doctors?

- Could change release resources to spend on other patients' healthcare needs, or would alternative systems be as, or more, expensive?

- Some patients are anaesthetised by trainee doctors in their first year in anaesthesia without direct supervision (Chapter 2). Is this more or less safe than being anaesthetised by an experienced and well-trained assistant who is under the supervision of a consultant immediately available within the theatre suite?

- Nurses monitor very ill patients who are being treated with multiple interventions in ICU; how does this compare in risk to monitoring a healthy patient undergoing a minor operation?

- An inability to recruit consultants, or staff an operating list when a consultant is absent, reduces the number of operations that some trusts can carry out (Chapters 1 and 2). Is it better for patients to wait untreated for their operation because of a lack of anaesthetists, or be treated by non-medically trained staff supervised by consultants within the theatre suite?

The service needs flexibility but the consultants' contract is not designed for it

Medical staff planning

160. To date, medical staffing policy has been dominated by planning at national and regional level that aims to increase the proportion of medical staff at consultant level, and regulate the number of trainee doctors to meet the demand for GPs and consultants. Most, if not all, trusts are also faced with changes that affect the demand for anaesthetists. These include changes to contracted activity, rationalisation of surgical services and reduction in trainees' contribution to services. Variations between trusts in the costs of anaesthetists, productivity, grade mix and supervision, suggest that some trusts can improve efficiency and economy through more systematic planning of their staffing needs.

161. Key questions that need to be addressed in staffing plans for anaesthetists are:

- how many anaesthetists are needed to deliver services?

- what is an appropriate grade mix for the type of work in the hospital?

- how can flexibility of staffing be increased so that services can respond quickly and efficiently to the demands placed on them?

Creating a more flexible anaesthesia service

162. Changes in staffing may have consequences for individual consultants' terms and conditions, and would need directorate and trust-wide support. For example, as the grade mix changes, consultants will need to be committed to the supervision of non-consultant career grade doctors and staff development. Clinical directors will need support from the medical director and chief executive to help foster this type of change.

163. This report has shown wide variation between trusts in the costs of anaesthetists, productivity, grade mix and supervision. Changes in arrangements for medical staffing can help to reduce this variation:

- greater flexibility is needed in job design – for example, to attract and retain doctors who do not want to work full-time, and who are trying to combine a career with bringing up a family;

- diversification is needed in the type of doctors who are employed – for example, more staff grade anaesthetists can be employed when the work does not require the skills of a consultant; and

- better management of the rota is needed and more flexibility in arrangements for covering consultants' absences.

164. But there is a more fundamental problem. There is a growing awareness of a conflict that is built into the system – the service needs flexibility, but the consultants' contract is not designed for it. Consultants' contracts fix the majority of their work to specific times and locations. This has the advantage of clarifying when each individual should attend, which is especially important when resources across the hospital will be committed (a surgical list involves not only the anaesthetist's costs, but also those of surgeons and theatre staff, of staff managing the waiting list, of theatre space, and for patients themselves).

165. But the disadvantage of a typical consultant's contract is that it discourages flexibility in covering absences or when new operating lists are created. Consideration should be given to how the current contract could be developed to promote greater flexibility in deployment. For most of the time consultants would still work a regular pattern because that is the nature of the work, but change would allow greater flexibility around the margins. This change needs to be considered at national level.

166. Finally, it is important to remember that 75 per cent of anaesthetists' costs are spent supporting surgery. Anaesthesia costs are rising in response to demand created by others, and over which anaesthetists do not have control. To solve future anaesthesia staffing problems, trusts will not only have to take action within the anaesthesia directorate, but also consider aspects of their service strategy that go beyond the specialty of anaesthesia.

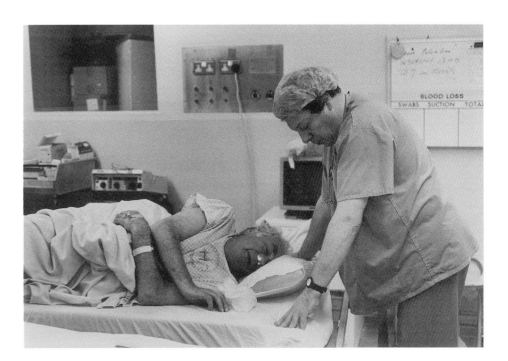

RECOMMENDATIONS

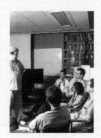

5 Leadership and Change

The recommendations follow the order in which they are discussed in the text. Priority recommendations are highlighted.

	Recommendation	Action needed by
1	Review the time and support needed to manage directorates effectively.	**Chief executive**
2	Align budgetary responsibility with those responsible for expenditure (for example, anaesthetic drugs and agents).	**Chief executive, clinical director, individual anaesthetists**
3	Decide on the appropriate limits of clinical freedom – for example, what to do if good practice guidelines agreed by the trust are not followed.	**Trust board, medical director, individual clinicians**
4	Sponsor research on whether the demand for doctors can be reduced, and the best use made of consultants' time, by allowing others who are appropriately trained to monitor/maintain anaesthesia without a medically qualified anaesthetist continually present in the operating room – for example, via carefully controlled pilot schemes.	**NHS Executive**
5	Develop a longer-term medical staff plan which should predict expected demand changes and show how these will be covered while ensuring supervision and solo opportunities for trainees.	**Medical director, clinical director**

Appendix 1

Acknowledgements

The advisory group

Dr Leslie Baird	President, the Association of Anaesthetists of Great Britain and Ireland
Dr Nicholas Bishop	Medical Director, Brighton Health Care NHS Trust, and the British Association of Medical Managers
Mr David Edgar	Business Manager of Theatres and Critical Care, Leicester Royal Infirmary
Mr Michael Edgar	Royal College of Surgeons
Sir Terence English	Audit Commissioner
Dr Peter Evans	Clinical Director, Anaesthetic Services, Charing Cross Hospital
Ms Rosalie Everatt	Director of Pain Wise UK
Sir Peter Kemp	Audit Commissioner
Mr Danny McCormack	Service Manager Anaesthetics, Basildon and Thurrock General Hospitals Trust, and British Association of Operating Department Assistants
Dr Mike McGovern	Health Care Directorate, NHS Executive
Ms Wilma McPherson	Director of Quality and Nursing, Guy's and St Thomas' Hospitals Trust
Dr Jean Millar	Consultant anaesthetist, Oxford Radcliffe Trust
Professor Cedric Prys-Roberts (from April 1997, Professor Leo Strunin)	President, Royal College of Anaesthetists
Ms Hilary Rowland	Audit Commissioner
Dr David Salter	Welsh Office
Mrs Helena Shovelton	Audit Commissioner
Sir Ron Watson	Audit Commissioner

Interview and data collection sites

We are grateful to the following trusts that gave of their time for interviews and/or assisted with data collection:

Basildon and Thurrock General Hospital NHS Trust
Bromley Hospitals NHS Trust
Burton Hospitals NHS Trust
Cardiothoracic Centre Liverpool NHS Trust
Central Manchester Healthcare Trust
Central Middlesex Hospital NHS Trust
Chelsea and Westminster Healthcare NHS Trust
Chesterfield/North Derbyshire Royal Hospital NHS Trust
Darlington Memorial Hospital NHS Trust
Eastbourne Hospitals NHS Trust
Freeman Group of Hospitals NHS Trust
Frenchay Healthcare NHS Trust
Gloucester Royal NHS Trust
Gwynedd Hospitals NHS Trust

Heatherwood and Wexham Park Hospital NHS Trust
Hereford Hospitals NHS Trust
Huddersfield NHS Trust
Kings Mill Centre for Health Care Services NHS Trust
Lewisham Hospitals NHS Trust
Llanelli/Dinefwr NHS Trust
Luton and Dunstable Hospital NHS Trust
Mid Cheshire Hospitals Trust
Mid Staffordshire General Hospitals NHS Trust
North Glamorgan NHS Trust
North Hertfordshire NHS Trust
North Staffordshire Hospital NHS Trust
Northampton General Hospital NHS Trust
Northern Devon Healthcare NHS Trust
Northwick Park & St Marks NHS Trust
Pain Research Unit, Oxford Radcliffe Hospital NHS Trust
Pontefract Hospitals NHS Trust
Portsmouth Hospitals NHS Trust
Preston Acute Hospitals NHS Trust
Princess Alexandra Hospital NHS Trust
Queen Mary's Sidcup NHS Trust
Queen's Medical Centre University Hospital NHS Trust
Royal Brompton Hospital NHS Trust
Royal Hull Hospitals NHS Trust
Royal Liverpool Children's Hospital NHS Trust
Royal Wolverhampton Hospitals NHS Trust
St Albans and Hemel Hempstead NHS Trust
St James and Seacroft University Hospitals NHS Trust
Salisbury Health Care NHS Trust
South Devon Healthcare NHS Trust
South Manchester University Hospitals NHS Trust
South Tees Acute Hospitals NHS Trust
Southampton University Hospitals NHS Trust
Southport and Formby NHS Trust
United Bristol Healthcare NHS Trust
United Leeds Teaching Hospitals NHS Trust
University Hospital of Wales Healthcare Trust
West Cumbria Health Care NHS Trust
West Dorset General Hospitals NHS Trust
West Suffolk Hospitals NHS Trust
Wirral Hospital NHS Trust

Others sites

We are grateful for informal discussions with many other clinicians and managers, and with local auditors. Many anaesthetists have given a considerable amount of their time in ensuring that the study team have had access to information.

Appendix 2

Data sources

National surveys

Audit Commission survey of consultant anaesthetist shortages

A three-page questionnaire was sent to every acute trust director of personnel in the UK in June 1997. The questionnaire asked for the number of vacant posts, expenditure on locums, and whether any problems were easing or increasing. The survey aimed to provide a national picture of where shortages occur and the methods that trusts have used to try to overcome them. A definitive response rate is difficult to state, because some trusts that we wrote to, but which did not reply, may be providing acute services without employing their own anaesthetists. However, the simple response rate based on the number of questionnaires mailed was 202 usable replies (69 per cent).

Audit Commission survey of maternity services

A short form was sent to every acute trust in England and Wales, addressed to the clinical director of anaesthesia. It asked for details of staff cover for the maternity unit, the number of consultant sessions, activity information about the number of caesarean section and other interventions, and the number of normal labour epidurals, etc. By the closing date, 138 forms had been returned, giving a likely response rate of 70 per cent. It is not certain that all the trusts that were mailed offered maternity services, although those writing back to say that they did not have been excluded from the response-rate calculation.

Audit Commission survey of pain after surgery

A seven-page questionnaire was sent to every acute trust chief executive in the UK in June 1997. The chief executive was asked to forward it for completion to a suitable person (for example, pain team head if one existed; otherwise the clinical director for surgery or anaesthesia), and return a tear-off slip notifying the Audit Commission of who had been asked to complete the form. The questions covered organisation; guidelines, training and audit; patient-controlled and epidural analgesia; patient activity statistics, and the existence and make-up of acute pain teams. The survey built on two previous surveys that had been carried out in 1994.

Where trusts were known to contain more than one separate acute hospital providing surgery of at least 80 beds, separate copies of the questionnaire were sent with a request to complete one for each hospital 'if they have quite separate services'. Trusts were asked to request extra copies if the number sent was incorrect, or to photocopy the original. Because there is no exact definition of what constitutes an acute hospital (the choice of 80 beds was an arbitrary one), there is no definitive list in existence. Exact response rates at hospital level are therefore unknown – 304 questionnaires were returned. Of the 291 trusts mailed to, 94 per cent returned at least one questionnaire.

NHS Executive data

Some nationally collected data were used – for example, information on outpatient consultations and follow-up appointments.

Surveys of day surgery patients' experiences in 43 self-selected hospitals

A questionnaire designed for the Audit Commission, described in *Measuring Quality: The Patient's View of Day Surgery* (HMSO, 1991), has been administered between 1991 and 1995 in 43 hospitals, with 11,053 patients returning questionnaires. The surveys have been conducted by the London School for Hygiene and Tropical Medicine, and the University of York (M Pettigrew, NHS Centre for Reviews and Dissemination).

Audit Commission study sites

Randomly selected subset of trusts

Forty-seven acute trusts were randomly selected and asked to take part in data collection between March and May 1997. Thirty-nine agreed to take part (listed in Appendix 1). The response rates for the different types of question varied, and are given separately at each point in the text. Thirty-nine completed returns for most aspects, an approximately 17 per cent sample of the acute trusts employing anaesthetists in England and Wales.

Interview study sites

These are listed in Appendix 1. Seven trusts were arbitrarily selected to present a range of problems – different areas of the country; small, medium and large trusts; teaching and non-teaching; some with known shortages of consultants, some without recruitment problems; etc. Many anaesthetists and managers were interviewed, and information collected during visits that lasted several days. In addition, a large number of trusts were visited for specific reasons – to discuss a particular problem or good practice approach.

Surveys of patients' experiences in interview study sites

At the seven interview study sites, patients leaving hospital during one week in July 1997 were given a self-completion questionnaire to take home with them. The questionnaire asked about who discussed their anaesthetic and pain relief with them before their operation, the information that they received, whether they had any pain and other after-effects. Separate questionnaires were prepared for inpatients and day surgery patients. Out of a total of 596 questionnaires distributed, 229 were returned for analysis, an overall response rate of 38 per cent. Response rates at the different trusts ranged from 26 to 60 per cent.

Appendix 3

Cost component tree and definitions

Cost component tree

The overall cost of anaesthetising patients is broken down into the different component parts, and the most important are analysed in the text of the report. This tree explains their inter-relations.

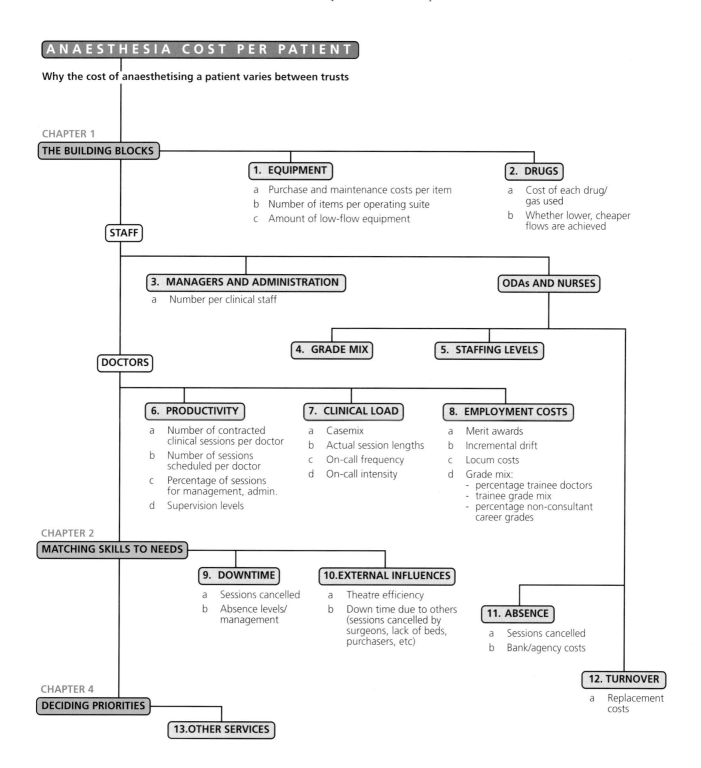

ANAESTHESIA COST PER PATIENT

Why the cost of anaesthetising a patient varies between trusts

CHAPTER 1
THE BUILDING BLOCKS

1. EQUIPMENT
a   Purchase and maintenance costs per item
b   Number of items per operating suite
c   Amount of low-flow equipment

2. DRUGS
a   Cost of each drug/gas used
b   Whether lower, cheaper flows are achieved

STAFF

3. MANAGERS AND ADMINISTRATION
a   Number per clinical staff

ODAs AND NURSES

4. GRADE MIX

5. STAFFING LEVELS

DOCTORS

6. PRODUCTIVITY
a   Number of contracted clinical sessions per doctor
b   Number of sessions scheduled per doctor
c   Percentage of sessions for management, admin.
d   Supervision levels

7. CLINICAL LOAD
a   Casemix
b   Actual session lengths
c   On-call frequency
d   On-call intensity

8. EMPLOYMENT COSTS
a   Merit awards
b   Incremental drift
c   Locum costs
d   Grade mix:
   - percentage trainee doctors
   - trainee grade mix
   - percentage non-consultant career grades

CHAPTER 2
MATCHING SKILLS TO NEEDS

9. DOWNTIME
a   Sessions cancelled
b   Absence levels/management

10. EXTERNAL INFLUENCES
a   Theatre efficiency
b   Down time due to others (sessions cancelled by surgeons, lack of beds, purchasers, etc)

11. ABSENCE
a   Sessions cancelled
b   Bank/agency costs

12. TURNOVER
a   Replacement costs

CHAPTER 4
DECIDING PRIORITIES

13. OTHER SERVICES

Cost component definitions

The different indicators taken from the tree and displayed in separate exhibits are defined in the following list:

Definitions

EXHIBIT 3: Cost per clinical session

Salary costs:

- consultants and associate specialists multiplied by 10/11 to calculate maximum part-time salary from whole-time equivalent salary; and

- grade mid-points are used – the actual cost to each trust will vary according to incremental point distributions and merit awards, plus employers' add-on costs.

Sessions:

- the number of clinical sessions on the template rota.

EXHIBIT 5: Productivity

Staffing WTE from 1997/98 budget statements, including trainees at 100 per cent.

EXHIBIT 6: Job plans by trust

Includes only consultants with a whole-time or maximum part-time contract, and excludes anaesthetists with non-clinical fixed commitments.

EXHIBIT 7: Session lengths

Excludes sessions officially designated as all-day, but it is not known how many of the very long sessions in this exhibit are recognised in job plans by more than one half-day.

EXHIBIT 15: Theatre staff

Includes ODAs, nurses, support workers and other related staff, and are for funded posts at actual pay-bands relating to the main grades.

EXHIBIT 18: Cover

Cover by consultants in sample weeks at different times of the year, specified by the Audit Commission, are based on weekly plans produced in advance. It is possible that some consultants were not in fact present as planned, or alternatively an expected absence may not have occurred. On balance, the exhibit is likely to somewhat underestimate true absence levels.

EXHIBIT 19: Temporary theatre staff

Theatre staff definition as for **EXHIBIT 15**.

EXHIBIT 20: Cancelled sessions

A cancellation was defined as a session that had been scheduled, but then did not take place. Respondents were also asked to state whether the trust was unable to schedule some sessions in the first place due to staff shortages or other reasons and, if possible, to estimate the number. Data were supplied by theatre managers either for the whole year 1996/97; or a specified series of eight weeks spread throughout the year; or, if not collected standardly, from any audit period used by the trust. There was no tendency for the different sample periods to produce systematically different cancellation rates or reasons, and thus data from all trusts have been combined for the exhibit.

EXHIBIT 23: Visits

The questionnaire asked consultants to reply with regard to their most recent afternoon and morning operating lists. There was no difference in pattern between the two, so they have been combined for the exhibit.

CASE STUDY 6: Cost of pain control

TABLE 3: Chronic pain clinics

The same three time periods as described for Exhibit 21 were used, and again no systematic difference appeared between them. 'Other' reasons include planned place of discharge in fact not available, planned escort home not available, etc.

These are staff who have a regular sessional commitment to the clinic, rather than simply a referral arrangement.

Planned and actual work

The main cost estimates used in the report are based on the scheduled sessions listed in the 'template rota' that were collected from trusts which produce one. This shows the surgical and other sessions planned for each weekday morning and afternoon, together with the name of the anaesthetist usually fixed to each. It also lists the on-call arrangements for covering the 24-hour period. These rota reflect the usual pattern of work throughout the year, and are relatively straightforward and cheap to analyse. The template rota should reflect consultants' job plans. For the most part they do, but not in all trusts; thus, the template rota is a more reliable indicator of actual workloads and costs.

Casemix and complexity definitions

Although the 'ASA score' of a patient is not designed for assessing anaesthesia risk, it is widely used. But this is far from a comprehensive measure of the difficulty and risk of anaesthetising a patient. NCEPOD recommended in 1993 that 'some matching between ASA status and the skill (qualifications and [or] experience) of the anaesthetist deployed should be attempted by departments'. The Audit Commission model develops the concept of relating skills deployed to the complexity of work. It is time-consuming for anaesthetists to record all the details necessary to arrive at a better measure of difficulty and risk, but we are grateful to those study sites that did do so for every patient who was anaesthetised during one sample week.

Similar work is under development by the Society for Computing and Technology in Anaesthesia (SCATA). Their 'relative values' model measures anaesthetists' workload in terms of effort (time) and skill (complexity of the case). SCATA has collected data about the time spent by anaesthetists at routine operations, but as yet no data have been collected to validate the factors chosen to measure case complexity, and the model is a subject of current debate. The Audit Commission model uses similar factors to define case complexity and can be applied to urgent and emergency cases as well as to routine work. The validity of the model has been checked with the help of seven anaesthetists who gave advice, independently of one another, on the specification of the model and weightings used in it. The model has been tested at eight trusts and will be applied at more during local audits in 1998.

The following variables were recorded and used as proxy measures of the complexity and risk of the anaesthetic episode and of the skill and ability needed by the anaesthetist to deliver safe and efficient care:

- **ASA status of the patient** (1, 2, 3, 4 or 5)
- **Age of the patient** (< 3 months, >3 months, <3 years, >3 years, <10 years, <10 years < 65 years, <65 years)
- **Anaesthetic technique** (type of anaesthesia, airway management, ventilation, infusion of intravenous fluids, invasive monitoring)
- **Urgency of the operation** (routine, urgent, emergency).

Scores are applied to each of the subcategories of the factors. ASA status, age of the patient and anaesthetic technique have equal weight, with maximum possible scores of 16. The maximum score for urgency of the operation is 12. Operations are classified into one of four bands of complexity: low, medium, high and very high, according to their cumulative score. The bands are based on survey results from a reference trust (a teaching hospital) which displayed the full range of scores from low to very high:

Band	Reference trust
Low	25 per cent of operations with lowest complexity
Medium	Next 50 per cent of operations (in the inter-quartile range, 25 per cent to 75 per cent)
High	Next 20 per cent of operations above the upper quartile
Very high	5 per cent of operations with highest complexity

Appendix 4

Operating theatre efficiency

It is of little use a trust employing a cost-effective number and mix of anaesthetists if factors outside their control stop them working efficiently. The most obvious example is when trusts are trying to meet surgical contract demands: the efficiency with which operating theatres run directly affects anaesthetist productivity. Theatre efficiency was the subject of intense study at the end of the 1980s, and there is no lack of material setting out good practice in managing operating theatres (Ref. 97). But many trusts still suffer inefficiencies in their surgical processes [BOX J].

The keys to operating theatre efficiency extend well beyond the walls of the theatre suite – the research for this study identified over one hundred problems at different stages of the process, including aspects as diverse as a lack of surgical beds, poor management of theatre time or slow delivery of patients to theatre by porters, in addition to the way in which anaesthetists themselves work. The text considers the factors that involve anaesthetists.

BOX J

Operating theatre utilisation

Theatre efficiency is influenced at a range of levels, from trust management down to the specific way in which individual theatres are used day-to-day. External audits at more than 70 hospitals found that half of all theatres still do not reach the 90 per cent utilisation target set by the Bevan Report of 1989. On average, audits identified scope for increasing the number of patients treated by 10 per cent for the same expenditure, or equivalent savings. There are wide differences in expenditure on staff per theatre session, and in the number of patients operated on per session, even within specialties where casemix is similar. In addition, the National Performance Advisory Group (NPAG) has begun a process of benchmarking theatre performance. Its first report, based on results from 20 hospitals, has just been issued. It covers planned and cancelled operating hours for both elective and emergency patients, session under and over-runs, and theatre staff costs. Annual updates are planned.

What affects efficiency? The views of working surgeons, anaesthetists and theatre managers

The majority of surgeons, anaesthetists and managers at two trusts thought that their theatres were fairly efficient, but one in five thought there was room for substantial improvement. When asked to rate 50 factors that might affect theatre efficiency, they rated the following as most important. The reasons are listed in order of how many people think them important; only a few directly involve the way in which anaesthetists and the staff work with them behave:

cont./

BOX J (cont.)

Factors that limit efficiency

- emergency cases pushing into elective lists, causing elective cancellations or delays;
- sessions starting late enough to cause a patient to be cancelled from the list, or fewer patients to have been scheduled for the list than could have been (can be caused by anaesthetists or support staff, but more usually by surgeons, according to respondents);
- sessions over-running enough to create problems for the following list;
- delays because some patients are not ready for theatre when required;
- portering delays in bringing patients to theatre or taking them from recovery afterwards, causing bottlenecks;
- lack of intensive care beds or staff; and
- inexperienced theatre staff.

Things that have enhanced efficiency

- audit or consultancy project focusing attention on areas that need improvement;
- reviewing surgical contracts and re-allocating sessions between specialties to match;
- improving liaison between anaesthesia and surgical departments, reducing the number of sessions cancelled at short notice;
- improving cover arrangements, leading to fewer sessions being cancelled by anaesthetists;
- scheduled daytime emergency sessions;
- introducing pre-admission clinics, reducing patient 'no shows';
- system for contacting patients a few days in advance, or on the morning of surgery, allowing list substitutions to be invited from the waiting list;
- introducing anaesthetic checklists and guidelines, for completion by the patient, nurse or surgical team, reducing delays due to missing information; and
- appropriate major cases scheduled for the morning, allowing safe return to ward from recovery room without need for HDU/ICU.

Potential efficiency enhancers, introduced in some trusts, but yet to be tried in these

- introducing incentives/fines to reduce cancellations by surgical specialties or anaesthesia directorate;
- referral to specialty rather than individual surgeon, leading to more efficient list construction and fewer cancellations;
- theatre, anaesthesia and recovery staff cross-cover, reducing cancellations due to absence; and
- introducing three-session days, with the third session being a shorter shift that begins at 5pm.

BOX J (cont.)

Keeping on top of the problem

Theatres are dynamic places, and the flow of patients must be monitored constantly to ensure that future efficiency is optimised. This requires the attention of a person who is both able to spot developing crises and blockages, and has the authority to take action to prevent them stopping throughput; and an IT system that can provide statistics about cancellation rates and reasons, whether sufficient notification is being given and lists re-scheduled, etc. IT can also help to construct optimal theatre lists from patients on waiting lists that make the best use of resources. Even more improvement can be made if a hospital is able to introduce more radical changes – for example, monitoring of the state of each operating theatre, enabling on-the-day re-deployment of staff, cancelling the last patient if the list is likely to over-run, adding any suitable urgent cases if a list is under-running, etc. The most fundamental requirement for improvement is that doctors and theatre staff understand the importance of improved efficiency and the part that they can play in this, and a theatre manager with the ability to interpret these statistics who has the authority to make changes.

Source: Audit Commission site visits; District Audit, 'Despatch 2 on operating theatres', 1996

Appendix 5

Good quality written information for patients

Someone should be nominated as responsible for producing written information, and this person will need to consult all the different professions involved, as well as patients. Someone also needs to be responsible for ensuring supplies of the document(s), their distribution, and for informing new staff about use. Regular audit should check that patients receive the information, that they receive it at the right time, and whether they find it of help. Written information can be compared with this checklist:

Anaesthesia

Types of anaesthetic (general/local/etc) and how it will be administered	
Situations in which it may be clinically appropriate to offer a choice	
The role and effects of pre-medication	
Recovery period – what will happen and where	
Possible side-effects and what to do if you experience them	
Postoperative pain and pain relief	
What the aims of the hospital are in the relief of pain	
Likely pain type and levels you can expect after different types of operation	
What to do if you experience pain	
Going home	
What to do if you experience pain at home	
The prescription you are given	
Who to contact if you have concerns – someone at the hospital or your GP	

Source: Audit Commission

Appendix 6

Cost-effectiveness of chronic pain services

Evidence-based treatments

Chronic pain treatments are classified by evidence of effectiveness and the risk of side-effects, degree of invasiveness and cost of the procedure. The percentage of 20 trusts providing each treatment is listed where known; some treatments may be provided via referral to another clinic.

The effectiveness of some treatments has not been proved, some have a risk of side-effects or further damage and some are expensive. For these reasons, it makes sense that, generally speaking, treatment should begin with those in the lightest shaded boxes of the table and proceed to the darkest shaded boxes more rarely, based on individual clinical judgement, if other treatments are contra-indicated or have been found not to work.

Clinical risk and/or cost*	Evidence of effectiveness: Effective**	Thought to be effective, but with little formal evidence***	Ineffective****
Low	Some minor oral analgesics (for example, ibuprofen, paracetamol)	TENS provided for use at home 90%	Some minor oral analgesics (for example, codeine alone)
	Topical NSAIDs in rheumatological conditions (for example, single arthritic joint pain) 90%	Relaxation therapy	
	Topical capsaicin in diabetic neuropathy, psoriasis 95%		
Medium	Antidepressant drugs (for example, for neuropathic pain, post-herpetic neuralgia, diabetic neuropathy) 95%	Outpatient TENS courses 60%	Injection of corticosteroids in or around shoulder joints for shoulder pain 89%
	Anticonvulsant drugs (for example, for trigeminal neuralgia) 100%	Outpatient psychological intervention programmes 70%	
	Systemic local anaesthetic drugs for nerve injury pain 60%	Acupuncture courses by nurse or therapist 50%	
		Manipulation for back pain 50%	
		Epidural given once, but abandoned if ineffective	
		Long-term, low-rate opiates	
		Surgical intervention for back pain when surgery has not yet been tried (for example, laminectomy for sciatica with positive neurological signs and MRI)	
		Orthopaedic corsets, neck collars used for long periods	
		Sclerosing injection for low back pain 21%	

Clinical risk and/or cost*	Evidence of effectiveness: Effective**	Thought to be effective, but with little formal evidence***	Ineffective****
High	Epidural for back pain and sciatica (effects for first 60 days)	Acupuncture courses provided by doctors (higher salary costs) 65%	Epidural for back pain and sciatica (effects beyond 3 months)
	Inpatient psychological intervention programmes 25%	Trigeminal neuralgia treatments using specialised/expensive equipment (for example, radio frequency block kit) 30%	Intravenous regional sympathetic blockade with guanethidine 90%
		Lignocaine infusion as inpatient 45%	
		Epidural left in situ for several weeks as inpatient 84%	
		Long-term high doses of a cocktail of opiates and other drugs	
		Repeated back pain surgery	
		Cordotomy 11%	
		Spinal cord implanted stimulators 25%	
		Destructive nerve burning, freezing, phenol injections 95%	

* Treatments in medium or high categories may be rated thus on either clinical risk or cost, or both. Treatments classified as low are both low risk and cost. Clinical risks could include side-effects, the degree of invasiveness of the procedure, and whether the effects on the body are reversible. Treatments have been placed into a category according to the professional judgement of consulted practitioners.

** Treatments proved to be effective are those with a sufficient number of randomised control trials available to calculate a statistic called the 'number needed to treat' (NNT), and, in this context, which have values of NNT between 2 and 4.

*** Many treatments have not been subjected to enough randomised control trials to make a statistical judgement about their effectiveness.

**** Treatments shown to be without effect in this context are those with NNTs greater than 4.

Source: Audit Commission; evidence of effectiveness is drawn from Ref. 84; relative risk/cost from discussion with practitioners

Do chronic pain clinics reduce other NHS expenditure? A case study

At the request of the Audit Commission, one pain clinic carried out a preliminary study. A randomly selected group of 21 patients who first attended the clinic in October 1996 were asked to take part in a telephone interview. Some of the answers could be verified from clinic casenotes, but mostly the results are reliant on the patients' memories. The interviewer (an experienced research nurse) asked the patients about their consultation and treatment histories in the six months before attending the pain clinic, and in the six months since first attending, using a structured questionnaire. The main findings are:

- the number of consultations with other specialties did drop significantly (for example, with orthopaedic surgeons, general surgeons, etc), but the extra costs of attending the pain clinic offset this;

- the number of NHS treatments was also fewer, especially the more expensive options, but this was not a statistically significant reduction;

- there was no overall change in drug consumption; and

- the clinic covered its costs by reducing consumption elsewhere within the acute trust, and there were also cost savings to the NHS by significantly reduced GP consultations, while patients benefited from significantly reduced private treatment costs.

Average number per patient	In the six months Before pain clinic	After pain clinic	Change (+ = increase – = reduction)
Outpatient attendances			
NHS pain clinic	0.05	1.6	+97%*
Other NHS medical specialties**	2.8	0.9	-222%*
Total	2.8	2.5	-13%
NHS treatments (for example, TENS, physiotherapy, surgery)	1.0	0.9	-17%
Days in hospital	0.2	0.5	+50%
A/E attendances	0.1	0.05	-100%
Different types of drug for pain	2.0	2.2	+11%
Visits to the GP about pain	5.0	3.0	-64%*
Home visits by GP	0.1	0.1	-
Other NHS home visits	0	0	-
Private treatments	0.4	0.2	-125%*

Percentage of patients	Before	After
Attending outpatient clinics		
NHS pain clinic	5%	100%
Other NHS medical specialties**	81%	38%
Either	86%	100%
Having NHS treatment		
Relatively high cost treatments (for example, surgery)	10%	5%
Medium cost (for example, physiotherapy, nerve block)	62%	43%
Low cost (for example, x-ray)	24%	38%
Any treatment	67%	62%
Hospital inpatient	5%	10%
Attending A/E	5%	5%
Taking drugs for pain		
Opiates	14%	16%
Antidepressants, tranquillisers, etc	24%	47%
NSAIDs	48%	63%
Minor analgesics	71%	74%
Any type of drug	90%	90%
Visiting the GP about pain		
For repeat prescriptions	67%	52%
For consultation/advice about pain	62%	24%
Any reason to do with pain	86%	71%
Having a home visit by GP	5%	5%
Other NHS home visits	0%	0%
Having private treatment	33%	19%

* Significant change (paired sample t-test, 1-tailed, 5 per cent level).

** Other NHS specialties include orthopaedics, neurology, vascular surgery, gynaecology, urology, rehabilitation medicine, nephrology.

Glossary

AAGBI	Association of Anaesthetists of Great Britain and Ireland.
Anaesthesia	Derived from Greek and translated as 'without feeling'.
Anaesthetic agent	Drugs used to induce any aspect of anaesthesia (sleep, pain relief or relaxation).
Anaesthetic machine	These transport and supply anaesthetic gases from their source in cylinders or tanks, via flexible pipelines, through the machine to its outlet. Pressure regulators provide gases to flowmeters at a constant pressure. Pressure gauges indicate the pressure in the gas cylinder or the gas pipeline. Flowmeters are used to adjust the flow from the machine. After passing through the flowmeters, the gases mix and may be used to vaporise volatile anaesthetic agents before passing to the machine outlet. Suction apparatus is available to clear vomit from the respiratory tract.
Analgesia	Also from Greek and meaning 'without pain'.
Anti-emetic	A drug to counteract postoperative nausea.
ASA status	American Society of Anesthesiologists' (ASA) Classification of Physical Status for Anaesthesia:

ASA 1: The patient has no organic, physiological, biochemical or psychiatric disturbance. The pathological process for which operation is to be performed is localised and does not entail a systemic disturbance. Examples: a fit patient with inguinal hernia, fibroid uterus in an otherwise healthy woman.

ASA 2: Mild to moderate systemic disturbance caused either by the condition to be treated surgically or by other pathophysiological processes. Examples: non- or only slightly limiting organic heart disease, mild diabetes, essential hypertension, or anaemia. Some might choose to list the extremes of age here, either the neonate or the octogenarian, even where no discernible systemic disease is present. Extreme obesity and chronic bronchitis may be included in this category.

ASA 3: Severe systemic disturbance or disease from whatever cause, even though it may not be possible to define the degree of disability with finality. Examples: severely limiting organic heart disease, severe diabetes with vascular complications, moderate to severe degrees of pulmonary insufficiency, angina pectoris or healed myocardial infarction.

ASA 4: Severe systemic disorders that are already threatening life, not always correctable by operation. Examples: patients with organic heart disease showing marked signs of cardiac insufficiency, persistent angina, or active myocarditis, advanced degrees of pulmonary, hepatic, renal or endocrine insufficiency.

ASA 5: The moribund patient who has little chance of survival but is submitted to operation in desperation. Examples: burst abdominal aneurysm with profound shock, major cerebral trauma with rapidly increasing intracranial pressure, massive pulmonary embolus. Most of these patients require operation as a resuscitative measure with little if any anaesthesia.

Associate specialist	A doctor who is neither a consultant nor a trainee; although associate specialists have not completed a full course of anaesthesia training, they are often quite senior in skills and experience in some aspects of anaesthesia practice.
Breathing circuit	Breathing circuits deliver the gases from the anaesthetic machine outlet to the patient's lungs. Breathing circuits may be integral to the anaesthetic machine. There are three main types:

       1. open circuits, where gas is, for example, provided by a mask which is held clear of the face and where oxygen supply is derived from the room air, and where expired gases escape freely into the atmosphere;

       2. circuits with an adequate fresh gas flow that is sufficient for carbon dioxide elimination (Magill, Bain and Lack circuits are examples); and

       3. closed circuits with inadequate fresh gas flow which rely on soda-lime for elimination of carbon dioxide. Oxygen is added to the system and the same anaesthetic mixture can be re-breathed over and over again (low-flow circuits).

Caesarean section	Childbirth where the baby is removed through a surgical incision in the abdomen, rather than by normal delivery. Because it is an operation, an anaesthetist will be present either to give a general anaesthetic, or to administer a spinal or epidural anaesthetic.
Calman	The Calman training requirements mean that there will be a time-limit on how long a trainee can spend at each stage. The aim is to improve the training process and make the supply of potential consultants easier to manage. The full reference to the report is given in the references section.
Cardiac-arrest or 'crash' team	Team of doctors and other staff who are on-call within the hospital to attend cardiac arrests.
Clinical assistant	A doctor who is neither a consultant nor a trainee; often a GP who has trained previously in anaesthesia (similar posts may be titled hospital practitioner, or part-time medical officer).
Closed circuits	Circuit where gases are recycled through the anaesthetic machine and patient.
CPD	Continuing professional development.
Consultant	An independent medical practitioner whose name is entered on the specialist register of the General Medical Council (GMC), who is contracted to provide anaesthesia services for a trust, and who may provide training.
Elective patients	Patients whose attendance at hospital has been booked in advance.
Epidural	A continuous infusion of local anaesthetic via a catheter inserted into the patient's back, that numbs the area around the abdomen and back. Epidurals are often given for pain relief during childbirth, but are also used to control the pain of patients who have had major abdominal or thoracic surgery.
GA	General anaesthesia.
HDU	High dependency unit.
ICU, ITU	Intensive care unit, intensive therapy unit.

IM	Intramuscular.
Induction	Making the patient unconscious.
Intubation (extubation)	Insertion (removal) of a breathing tube into (from) a patient's windpipe.
IV	Intravenous.
LA	Local anaesthesia.
Laryngeal mask	A small mask on the end of a tube which sits on the laryngeal inlet.
Laryngoscope	Device used to pass an endotracheal tube into the larynx under direct vision.
Locum	A temporary doctor bought in as cover from an agency or another hospital; may be any grade.
Maintenance	Keeping unconscious.
Middle grade	Formerly a registrar (R) or senior registrar (SR); now a specialist registrar (SpR).
Monitor	A wide range of monitoring devices may be used during anaesthesia to record and warn of changes to heart rate, temperature, blood pressure, oxygen levels in the blood, etc.
MTO	Medical Technical Officer.
Muscle relaxant	A drug used to assist intubation, make abdominal or thoracic surgery easier/possible, or on occasion in the ICU for long-term ventilation.
NCEPOD	National Confidential Enquiry into Perioperative Deaths.
New Deal	The 'New Deal' on trainee doctors' hours of work is designed to reduce the number spent on duty in any one week. The full reference to the report is given in the references section.
NHD	Notional half-day.
NSAID	Non-steroidal anti-inflammatory drug.
NVQ	National vocational qualification.
ODA	Operating department assistant.
ODP	Operating department practitioner.
Open circuit	Circuit with no re-breathing.
Operation classification according to degree of urgency	The most commonly used classification is that given in the NCEPOD reports:
	Emergency: Immediate lifesaving operation, resuscitation simultaneous with surgical treatment (for example, trauma, ruptured aortic aneurysm). Operation usually within one hour.
	Urgent: Operation as soon as possible after resuscitation (for example, irreducible hernia, intestinal obstruction, major fractures). Operation within 24 hours.
	Scheduled: An early operation but not immediately lifesaving (for example, malignancy). Operation usually within three weeks.
	Elective: Operation at a time to suit both patient and surgeon (for example, cholecystectomy, joint replacement).

OR	Operating room (theatre).
PCA	Patient-controlled analgesia.
PONV	Postoperative nausea and vomiting.
POP	Postoperative pain.
Premed, pre-medication	Sedation by drug and/or psychological anxiety-reduction before surgery.
PRHO	Pre-registration house officer.
RCA	Royal College of Anaesthetists.
Scrubbed	Theatre staff who have 'scrubbed up' to provide sterile operating conditions. They cannot therefore touch the outer packaging of the instruments, etc, used during the operation.
SHO	Senior house officer, the lowest grade of trainee doctor within most anaesthesia directorates.
SpR	Specialist registrar, the new term for the grade of trainee doctor above SHO.
Staff grade	A doctor who is neither a consultant nor a trainee. They have not completed a full course of anaesthesia training. They vary in skills and experience, but are often equivalent to a middle-grade trainee.
Syringe/infusion pump	Syringe and infusion pumps control the supply of fluids to a patient. A common use is the delivery of an intravenous agent for induction and maintenance of anaesthesia.
Template rota	A chart produced by the anaesthesia directorate, showing the surgical and other sessions planned for each weekday morning and afternoon, together with the name of the anaesthetist usually fixed to each. It also lists the on-call arrangements for covering the 24-hour period. These rota reflect the usual pattern of work throughout the year.
TENS	Transcutaneous nerve stimulation. Irritation of the skin overlying a painful area by a machine, used to alleviate pain.
Trust grade	Doctors with varying amounts of training and experience.
Volatile anaesthetic agents	Drugs usually used for maintenance of anaesthesia and sometimes induction.
WTE	Whole-time equivalent – a phrase used to describe calculations that express the hours of part-time employees as a proportion of a full-time post.

Notes

1. An estimate based on the annual Department of Health census of staff in post.

2. In this example the anaesthesia cost of a hernia repair operation was £74 (with a consultant anaesthetist both pre-assessing the patient and in the theatre, and at 1993 prices) (Ref. 99).

3. Although estimating the number needed to be deployed against each surgical session is easy (usually one to one), translating that into the required establishment, when a new surgeon is appointed, is not. Trusts recruit less than a whole-time equivalent (WTE) anaesthetist to cover the operating lists created by each new surgeon appointed because surgeons have more outpatient clinic and ward work to do. For example, one trust that was visited recruits either 0.56 or 0.74 WTE anaesthetists per 1 WTE surgeon, depending on whether the surgeon is contracted to do three or four operating lists a week. By contrast, a second trust budgets for only one-third of an anaesthetist for every new surgeon. Because few potential appointees wish to work a one-third part-time contract, cover is difficult until a second or third surgeon is appointed. In addition, there is no automatic trainee funding to accompany the consultant anaesthetist, making covering absences more difficult. (Source for second trust: Ernst & Young local value-for-money audit report, 1994/95.)

4. See Note 3. Figures given are for the main surgical specialties combined. The growth figures for all grades of staff are 27 per cent for anaesthetists, and 23 per cent for surgeons.

5. NHS Executive statistics. If emergency admissions continue to result in elective cancellations, there is a case for expecting the demand for anaesthetists and operating theatre staff to fall, since while 85 per cent or more of cancelled elective work is surgical, only half of emergency admissions require surgery. But in practice there has been no staff lay-off to date; most trusts appear to work over-capacity with the amount of emergency surgery cancelling out any reduced elective work.

6. One study has estimated the increased cost in staff needed to offset service reductions resulting from the Calman proposals to time-limit specialist training as 6 per cent of trust income (Ref. 6).

7. Regional Task Force returns for 31 March 1997, NHS Executive; the 80 per cent performance in anaesthesia compares with an average 77 per cent across all specialties. During the Audit Commission study, trainee doctors' self-reported hours differ from this – more than 50 per cent claimed to be working in excess of 56 hours, excluding rest times and lunch breaks (trainee survey across 42 trusts).

8. There is a significant difference in the distribution of commitments between the groups (chi squared = 23.7, df = 4, p < 0.001). Excludes clinical directors, etc, and part-timers. Source: Audit Commission, results for 300 consultants from 40 trusts.

9. The Association of Anaesthetists recommend auditing the average time that is taken in fulfilling fixed commitments to help determine how many NHDs the workload is equivalent to (Ref. 8). There have been occasional self-report diary exercises, although these have not been verified by direct observation. For example, in an exercise carried out in 1989, 79 consultant anaesthetists reported spending an average of 36 hours per week on NHS clinical work, plus another three hours in the hospital while on-call, and a further nine hours on other NHS activities such as teaching, management, administration, audit, etc – a total of 48 hours. This was similar to the average for all specialties. The variation between different anaesthetists and hospitals was not reported (Ref. 11).

10. First year trainees will require more supervision, while some specialties will need a greater proportion of training lists than routine surgical work (Ref. 12).

11. The ratio of trainees to consultants in 1993 was 1:1 in anaesthesia, the highest of the hospital specialties; the surgical specialties average at about 1.5:1, ranging from 1.3:1 in ophthalmology to 2.5:1 in obstetrics and gynaecology (Department of Health Medical Manpower Statistics, reported in Ref. 9).

12. Source: Royal College of Anaesthetists' annual statistics on consultant and staff grade appointments.

13. There is no central requirement for trusts to provide time for non-consultant career grade doctors to undertake CPD. Non-consultant career grade staff responding to Audit Commission questionnaires reported varying uptake of CPD: 46 per cent gained between 26-50 during 1995/96, 21 per cent more, and the remainder fewer; 9 per cent took more than 10 days study leave, 31 per cent 5-10 days, 29 per cent 1-5 days, and 32 per cent none (replies from 106 respondents across 40 trusts).

14. $r=0.48$, $N=20$, $p<0.05$.

15. ODAs – often, but not necessarily, trained to NVQ level 3 in Operating Department Practice – may work in the anaesthetic room, operating room or in recovery. Similarly, theatre nurses who have trained appropriately can work in the anaesthetic room or in recovery.

16. Further benefits may accrue if multi-skilled staff are grouped into teams by specialty. Teamworking potentially allows devolved decision-making at team leader level against objectives set by the theatre manager, a more varied career structure, and a breaking down of previous rigid boundaries between ODAs and nurses. Teams may develop a sense of wanting to improve performance together and solve problems, and improve throughput because team members become accustomed to working together. They may develop better relationships with the smaller number of wards with which they become linked, helping to ensure that delays do not occur because patients are either not ready for surgery or not collected on time from recovery.

17. Based on updating to current average prices the range of equipment for one operating theatre and anaesthetic room listed in Ref. 1.

18. The exact guidelines differ according to the type of equipment.

19. List cancellations at a large teaching hospital by anaesthetists theoretically cost the trust £350,000 in lost income during one year, and this amount of money could cover the cost of employing more anaesthetists to reduce cancellations (Source: District Audit local value-for-money report, 1994/95). But the theoretical saving is based on cost-per-case calculations – first, trusts would need to ensure that this amount of income is truly being lost, since most contracts are in fact on a 'block' basis, and under-activity will not necessarily result in this amount of income being lost. Even if there is a real income loss in one year that could be stopped by employing more anaesthetists, the trust would next need to estimate whether in future years contract demand, and income, will be maintained at this level and not leave the newly appointed anaesthetists an under-utilised extra cost.

20. Using the system for defining anaesthesia complexity set out in Appendix 3, initial survey results show that the proportion of consultant in-hours operations classified as of low complexity varied from 25 to 70 per cent across eight trusts.

21. This feature has been the case in each of the four years published so far (1991/92 to 1994/95), with slight differences in the exact percentages each year (Refs. 27-30).

22. Source: Houghton K, 'Anaesthetic Department: Workload and Planning', unpublished MS, 1995.

23. Several recent surveys of doctors in different parts of the country have assessed attitudes towards the prospect of providing more in-hospital emergency cover. In one, two-thirds of consultant anaesthetists said that they would provide a resident on-call service, if compensated (Ref. 34). But in a second survey, about half of the anaesthetists said that they would consider more out-of-hours work, but many were vehemently opposed to this concept, suggesting that if this becomes necessary, a mechanism for opting in and out of involvement might be required (Ref. 35).

24. Of those consultant anaesthetists attending a management course held at the University of Keele in February 1997 whose trusts had introduced daytime emergency operating sessions, half reported that at least one consultant anaesthetist's job plan contained half-days for fixed commitments to cover these sessions.

25. Mortality directly attributable to anaesthesia is so rare that valid statistical comparison between trusts is not possible. Critical-incident reporting is voluntary at the moment, as part of trusts' risk management processes and, again, data are not properly comparable either between grades within a trust, or between different trusts. There is a strong case for keeping better records, but apart from the problem of compliance and accuracy, the classification of incidents is quite complex. It would be important to differentiate between random accidents, equipment failures, problems due to the patient's medical, psychological or social condition, and actual staff errors. Within the latter category, it would then be necessary to distinguish between incidents due to lack of skill, lack of training, the failure to learn from training, tiredness, failure to carry out the usual checks, failure to call for assistance, problematic regulations, etc, before lessons could be learnt about how to avoid their recurrence (for example, Ref. 37).

26. Source: Audit Commission interviews with patients. The Audit Commission has already reported in full on the issue of communicating with patients. General findings were that there is often not enough information, or that it is poorly written or not what the patient wants to know. When written information does exist, it is often not given at all, given too late, or in too rushed or confusing a manner (Ref. 38). The Royal College of Anaesthetists states that verbal and written information should be provided to patients preoperatively to enable them to make an informed decision about pain relief (Ref. 39). The Association of Anaesthetists is producing a booklet for patients about anaesthesia. The Royal College of Nursing has issued a leaflet that emphasises how patients need to assess their own pain and be active in asking staff for help in relieving it; it does not offer advice on likely pain levels after specific types of procedure, and some common unfounded fears (for example, about addiction if morphine is used) are not addressed (Ref. 40).

27. One-third of 92 patients in seven trusts (source: Audit Commission survey of patients).

28. A similar overall proportion was recently reported in a separate large-scale study of surgical patients (Ref. 44).

29. On occasions, increasing postoperative pain may be the presentation of a complication that may require a surgical training to recognise its relevance and importance. In such situations, it would be wrong to look for more effective pain control.

30. Postoperative nausea and vomiting are common after general anaesthesia and for some patients can be more distressing than pain. Between 20 and 30 per cent of patients can expect to suffer (for example, Refs. 51, 52). In 1992 the Welsh Office issued a health gain target to reduce the proportion of people suffering from nausea and vomiting after an operation to under 25 per cent by 1995, and under 10 per cent by 2002 (Ref. 53). Similar principles to those applying to pain should also apply to nausea and vomiting, although in many patients these are more difficult to prevent than pain (for example, Ref. 54).

31. There are significant differences between hospitals in patients' reported pain, whether significance is tested using parametric or non-parametric tests. Standard error bars are plotted for ease of visual interpretation.

32. Since there is no tendency for studies with larger sample sizes, or those published in peer-reviewed journals, to report lower pain scores, the data have been combined for this exhibit. People react to pain stimuli differently – there is no physiological measure that matches experienced pain: hence pain specialists use the phrase 'pain is what the patient says it is'. Research suggests that simple, subjective, measures of pain reported by patients are worthwhile indicators both of experienced pain levels and of the impact of treatment upon experienced pain (for example, Ref. 56).

33. An American study found that one-third of all adverse drug events were related to analgesia, and half of the preventable events involved misuse or malfunction of epidural pumps or PCAs (reported in 'When Things Go Wrong', *Bandolier*, volume 28, 1996).

34. A sequential study introducing various aspects of good practice in pain relief found that the introduction of pain scoring and an algorithm for nurses and trainee doctors to follow about appropriate timing of intra-muscular injections produced the most significant reductions in patients' pain scores (Ref. 67).

35. Source: 304 hospital replies to the Audit Commission's national survey of pain after surgery.

36. It has been estimated that a basic pain team consisting of one or two consultant sessions and one whole-time equivalent nurse costs the equivalent of £5 per patient or about 0.5 per cent of the total cost of a surgical patient's hospital treatment (Dr Harmer, pers. comm.).

37. Source: 304 hospital replies to the Audit Commission's national survey of pain after surgery.

38. In 1983 the average epidural rate was 17 per cent – this has now risen to 21 per cent (average of 138 trusts providing data for this study). Fewer than one in ten units had an anaesthetist available solely for maternity throughout the 24-hour period, and one-quarter had no provision for an anaesthesia service at any time of the day. This has now improved – half of trusts replying to this study provide resident 24-hour cover, and only a very few small units have no service at all.

39. For example, in a 2,000-birth unit with a caesarean rate of 12.5 per cent and normal-labour epidural rate of 17 per cent, anaesthetists are likely to attend 1.6 events per 24 hours, and 4 per 24 hours in a large unit of 5,000 births with the same intervention rates.

40. Eleven per cent of 1,000 people, representative of the general population who were telephoned in 1990, said that they suffered from chronic pain (Ref. 76); 30 per cent of disabled adults reported severe recurring pain which limited normal daily living (Ref. 77).

41. A larger 1990 survey of 177 UK clinics found that only 14 per cent had consultant sessions from specialties other than anaesthesia; one-quarter had some input from psychologists, and three-quarters from physiotherapists, although these did not necessarily attend clinics all the time (Ref. 80). In 1994 it was estimated that about 200 pain clinics were in existence, mostly provided by acute trusts (Ref. 81). Minimum standards issued by the International Association for the Study of Pain for multidisciplinary pain clinics require access to and regular interaction with at least three types of clinician, one of whom should be a psychiatrist or psychologist (Ref. 82). See also material on the website of the UK Pain Society (http://www.ncl.ac.uk/~nanaes/painsoc.html).

42. Anaesthetists taking part in a survey in 1989 reported that 25 per cent of their patients were 'much better' following attendance, and a further 17 per cent were 'helped slightly', leaving the majority of patients with the same pain problem that they presented with (Ref. 83).

43. Self-help groups also encourage programmes that aim to help people to live with their pain (for example, Refs. 75, 85).

44. Ref. 88, reported in Ref. 84. This Canadian study estimated that while patients who attended a specialist pain clinic cost the total healthcare system about $3,000 a year, this was $2,000 less than for those who had not been referred to a clinic, mainly because they spent less time in hospital as inpatients.

45. In a recent national survey of clinical directors from all specialties, most reported that they spent nearly double their contracted hours on management tasks; about half are contracted for one session, the other half for two or more. Half felt undervalued for their management contribution and were thinking of returning to full-time clinical duties (Ref. 92).

46. Source: for 22 Audit Commission study sites providing data, 68 per cent of the variance in anaesthetists' cost per session is explained by the relationship with sessions per whole-time equivalent anaesthetist.

47. The different systems found in Europe are described in Vickers MD, 'More Audit', *Today's Anaesthetist*, pp27-8, 1997. In the USA, nurse anaesthetists are independent practitioners, somewhat akin to a UK midwife. By contrast, in most European systems, the non-medically trained staff act as assistants to the anaesthetist, under their direct control. There is debate about the overall cost equation of using nurse anaesthetists. They are paid at a higher level than UK ODAs, and their training costs are higher – but both these costs are less than those for doctors. The overall cost saving depends on the balance between these factors and reduced doctor time. Some of the factors that need to be considered have been aired by the Association of Anaesthetists (Ref. 17). But research in the UK context is lacking. As an example, in one Netherlands hospital visited during the Audit Commission study, a consultant-level anaesthetist covered two theatres, double the productivity of the UK system. In the USA, ratios vary but often involve one nurse anaesthetist in each theatre, plus an anaesthesiologist across three operating rooms. In both countries, the non-physician anaesthetist does not work with a separate assistant, but is paid at a higher level than UK ODAs or anaesthetic nurses. Thus the basic saving is the difference between the non-physician anaesthetist salaries and doctors in the operating rooms, plus the extra cost of the doctor overseeing these rooms. Some countries – for example, Belgium – have one doctor per theatre as in the UK, but have reduced operating theatre staffing costs by having only one person carrying out both anaesthetic and surgical support roles. Any research into overall cost savings in any of these systems would also need to take into account the effect of the staffing system on overall operating speed and training costs.

48. In the USA, the only country with data available comparing nurse anaesthetists working alone with anaesthesiologists (doctors) working alone, no significant differences in mortality have been found – partly because deaths are so rare whoever administers anaesthesia. The only published studies are now 20 years old, and suffer from the confounding effect that nurse anaesthetists working alone are more likely to do so in small isolated hospitals where emergency back-up might be less readily available (Refs. 94, 95).

References

1. Department of Health, *Hospital, Public Health Medicine and Community Health Service Medical and Dental Staff in England 1986 to 1996*, Statistical Bulletin 1997/17, Department of Health, 1997.

2. UK Health Departments, Joint Consultants' Committee and Chairmen of Regional Health Authorities, *Hospital Medical Staffing: Achieving A Balance - Plan for Action*, Department of Health, 1987.

3. NHS Management Executive, *Junior Doctors, The New Deal: Working Arrangements for Hospital Doctors and Dentists in Training*, Department of Health, London, 1991.

4. Department of Health, *Hospital Doctors: Training for the Future - The Report of the Working Group on Specialist Medical Training* (the 'Calman Report'), Department of Health, London, 1993.

5. Royal College of Anaesthetists, *Specialist Training in Anaesthesia, Supervision and Assessment*, London, 1994.

6. Newchurch and Co & West Suffolk Hospitals NHS Trust, *Catalyst for Change*, Regional Medical Executive of Anglia and Oxford Regional Office, 1996.

7. Department of Health, *Consultants' Contracts and Job Plans*, HC(90)16, Department of Health, London, 1990.

8. Association of Anaesthetists, *Guidance on Contracts and Workload for Consultant Anaesthetists*, AAGBI, London, 1997.

9. Audit Commission, *The Doctor's Tale: The Work of Hospital Doctors in England and Wales*, HMSO, 1995.

10. Audit Commission, *The Doctor's Tale Continued: The Audits of Hospital Medical Staffing*, Audit Commission/HMSO, 1996.

11. Office of Manpower Economics, *Survey of the Work and Responsibilities of Consultants in the NHS*, Department of Health, 1989.

12. Royal College of Anaesthetists' training guides: *SHOs* (1995), *Specialist Registrar*, London, 1996.

13. NHS Executive, *A Working Draft to Develop a Quality Framework for HCHS Medical and Dental staff*, EL(97)35, Leeds, 1997.

14. Association of Anaesthetists, *Non-consultant Career Grade Anaesthetists*, AAGBI, London, 1993.

15. National Association of Health Authorities and Trusts, *Hospital and Community Health Services Medical Recruitment Survey*, NAHAT, Birmingham, 1996.

16. Wilson R & Allen P, 'Medical and Dental Staffing Prospects in the NHS in England and Wales 1993', *Health Trends*, 26(3):70-9, 1994.

17. Association of Anaesthetists, *Anaesthesia in Great Britain and Ireland: A Physician-only Service*, AAGBI, London, 1996.

18. Harvey J et al, 'Project Has Been Set Up to Explore Ways of Preventing Wastage of Doctors', *BMJ*, 313:491, 1996; *BMJ*, 314:1591-2, 1996.

19. NHS Executive, *The Management and Utilisation of Operating Departments: The Bevan Report*, NHS Executive, 1989.

20. NHS Executive, VFM Update, 1995 issue 16.

21. Reilly C et al, *Professional Roles in Anaesthetics: A Scoping Study*, NHS Executive, Leeds, 1996.

22. Association of Anaesthetists, *Anaesthetic-related Equipment*, AAGBI, London, 1994.

23. Audit Commission, *Goods For Your Health*, Audit Commission, 1997.

24. Shepherd, M & Hanson, L, 'Kicking the Habit', *Health Service Journal*, 28 August 1997, pp28-9.

25. Cotter et al, 'Low-flow Anaesthesia: Practice, Cost Implications and Acceptability', *Anaesthesia*, 46:1009-12, 1991.

26. Audit Commission, *Finders, Keepers: The Management of Staff Turnover in NHS Trusts*, Audit Commission, 1997.

27. Campling E A, Devlin H B, Hoile R W, Lunn J N, *Report of the National Confidential Enquiry into Perioperative Deaths 1991/92*, NCEPOD, London, 1993.

28. Campling E A, Devlin H B, Hoile R W, Lunn J N, *Report of the National Confidential Enquiry into Perioperative Deaths 1992/93*, NCEPOD, London, 1995.

29. Campling E A, Devlin H B, Hoile R W, Lunn J N, *Report of the National Confidential Enquiry into Perioperative Deaths 1993/94*, NCEPOD, London, 1996.

30. Gallimore, S C, Hoile R W, Ingram, G S, Sherry, K M, *Report of the National Confidential Enquiry into Perioperative Deaths 1994/95*, NCEPOD, London, 1997.

31. Campling, E A, Devlin, H B, Hoile, R W, Ingram, G S, Lunn, J N, '*Who Operates When?*': A Report by the National Confidential Enquiry into Perioperative Deaths 1995/96, NCEPOD, London, 1997.

32. Audit Commission, *United We Stand*, Audit Commission/HMSO, London, 1996.

33. Royal College of Anaesthetists, *Specialist Training in Anaesthesia, Supervision and Assessment*, London, 1994.

34. Haldane G & Morrison A, 'Anaesthetists and the Calman Proposals', *Anaesthesia*, 52:181-2, 1997.

35. Dempsey G A & Skinner A, 'Attitudes of Consultant Anaesthetists to the Calman Proposals: A Questionnaire Survey', *Anaesthesia*, 51:975-7, 1996.

36. Derrington M C & Gallimore S, 'The Effect of the National Confidential Enquiry into Perioperative Deaths on Clinical Practice', *Anaesthesia*, 52:3-8, 1997.

37. Runciman W B et al, 'Errors, Incidents and Accidents in Anaesthetic Practice', *Anaesthetics and Intensive Care*, 21:506-19, 1993.

38. Audit Commission, *What Seems To Be The Matter: Communication Between Hospitals and Patients*, HMSO, London, 1993.

39. Royal College of Anaesthetists, *Guidance to Purchasers*, RCA, London, 1994.

40. Royal College of Nursing, *Pain Control After Surgery: A Patient's Guide*, London, RCN, 1996.

41. Vyvyan, H A L & Hanafiah Z, 'Patients' Attitudes to Rectal Drug Administration', *Anaesthesia*, 50: 983-4, 1995.

42. McQuay H, Moore A & Justins D, 'Treating Acute Pain in Hospital', *BMJ*, 314: 1531-5, 1997.

43. Mitchell J, 'A Fundamental Problem of Consent', *BMJ*, 310:43-8, 1995 (and following commentaries).

44. Bruster S et al, 'National Survey of Hospital Patients', *BMJ*, 309:1542-9, 1994.

45. Hayward, J, *Information: A Prescription Against Pain*, Royal College of Nursing, London, 1975.

46. Hathaway D, 'Effect of Preoperative Instruction on Postoperative Outcomes: A Meta-analysis', *Nursing Research*, 35:269-75, 1986.

47. Walding M F, 'Pain, Anxiety and Powerlessness', *Journal of Advanced Nursing*, 16:388-97, 1991.

48. Devine, E C, 'Effects of Psycho-educational Care for Adult Surgical Patients: A Meta-analysis of 191 Studies', *Patient Education and Counselling*, 19:127-42, 1992.

49. Fischer H B & Scott P V, 'Work Is Needed to Show that Good Quality Analgesia Improves Outcome of Surgery', *BMJ*, 311:1023-4, 1995.

50. Series of letters about postoperative pulmonary complications in *BMJ*, 312:1158-60, 1996.

51. Watcha M F & White P F, 'Postoperative Nausea and Vomiting: Its Aetiology, Treatment and Prevention', *Anaesthesiology*, 77:162-84, 1992.

52. Koivuranta M et al, 'A Survey of Postoperative Nausea and Vomiting', *Anaesthesia*, 52:443-9, 1997.

53. Welsh Health Planning Forum, *Protocol for Investment in Health Gain: Pain, Discomfort and Palliative Care*, Welsh Office: NHS Directorate, 1992.

54. Rowbotham D J, 'Current Management of Postoperative Nausea and Vomiting', *British Journal of Anaesthesia*, 69 (supplement): 46-59, 1992.

55. Working Party of the Commission on the Provision of Surgical Services, *Pain After Surgery*, Royal College of Surgeons & College of Anaesthetists, London, 1990.

56. Jenkinson C et al, 'Comparison of the Sensitivity to Change of Long and Short Term Pain Measures', *Quality of Life Research*, 4: 353-7, 1995.

57. Lehmann K A, 'New Developments in Patient-controlled Postoperative Analgesia', *Annals of Medicine*, 27:271-82, 1995.

58. Taylor N M Hall, GM & Salmon P, 'Patients' Experiences of Patient-controlled Analgesia', *Anaesthesia*, 51:525-8, 1996.

59. Gabrielczyk M R, and McGonagle C, 'Postoperative Pain Control: Influence of a Dedicated Acute Pain Nurse', *Anaesthesia*, 52: 382-94, 1997.

60. Hall G M, 'Patient-controlled Analgesia: Who Benefits?', *Anaesthesia*, 52:401-2, 1997.

61. Hawkshaw D, 'A Day Surgery Patient Telephone Follow-up Survey', *British Journal of Nursing*, 3:348-50, 1994.

62. Wilkinson D, Bristow A, Higgins D, 'Morbidity Following Day Surgery', *Journal of One-Day Surgery*, 2:5-6, 1992.

63. Marquardt H M, Razis P A, 'Prepacked Take-home Analgesia for Day Case Surgery', *British Journal of Nursing*, 5:1114-18, 1996.

64. Haynes T K, Evans D E and Roberts D, 'Pain Relief After Day Surgery: Quality Improvements by Audit', *Journal of One-Day Surgery*, pp12-15, Summer 1995.

65. Field L, 'Are Nurses Still Underestimating Patients' Pain Postoperatively?', *British Journal of Nursing*, 5:778-84, 1996.

66. Sofaer B, 'Pain Management Through Nurse Education', in Copp, L A (ed), *Perspectives On Pain*: Recent Advances in Nursing, 11, Churchill Livingstone, Edinburgh, 1985.

67. Gould T H et al, 'Policy for Controlling Pain After Surgery: Effect of Sequential Changes in Management', *BMJ*, 305:1187-93, 1992.

68. Wheatley R G et al, 'The First Year's Experience of an Acute Pain Service', *British Journal of Anaesthesia*, 67:353-9, 1991.

69. Goldhill D R, 'Introducing the Postoperative Care Team', *BMJ*, 314: 389, 1997; replies in *BMJ*, 314: 1346, 1997.

70. Windsor A L M, Glynn C J & Mason D G, 'National Provision of Acute Pain Services', *Anaesthesia*, 51:228-31, 1996.

71. Harmer M, Davies K A & Lunn J N, 'A Survey of Acute Pain Services in the United Kingdom', *BMJ*, 311:360-1, 1995.

72. Humphries C A et al, 'Audit of Prescribing: The Effect of Hospital Guidelines', *Anaesthesia*, 52: 745-9.

73. Department of Health et al, *Report on Confidential Enquiries Into Maternal Deaths in the UK 1991-1993*, HMSO, London, 1996.

74. Obstetric Anaesthetists Association, *Recommended Minimum Standards for Obstetric Anaesthesia Services*, Nottingham, 1995.

75. Everatt R, *An Introduction to Self-help Pain Management*, Pain Wise UK, Whitstable, 1996.

76. Rigge M, 'Pain', *Which? Way to Health*, April 1990, 66-8.

77. Astin M, Lawton D & Hirst M, 'The Prevalence of Pain in a Disabled Population', *Society of Scientific Medicine*, 42:1457-64, 1997.

78. Centre for Health Economics, *Back Pain: Its Management and Cost to Society*, York University, 1995.

79. McQuay H, Machin L & Moore R A, 'Chronic Non-malignant Pain: A Population Prevalence Study', *Practitioner*, 229:1109-11, 1985.

80. College of Health, *Pain Relief Clinics in the UK*, London, 1990.

81. College of Health, *The Pain Clinic Directory 1994*, College of Health, London, 1994.

82. Loeser J D, 'Desirable Characteristics for Pain Treatment Facilities: Report of the IASP Taskforce', in Bond, M R, Charlton, J E & Woolf, C J (eds), *Proceedings of the VIth World Congress on Pain*, Elsevier Science, BV, 1991.

83. Association of Anaesthetists, Royal College of Anaesthetists and Pain Society, *Anaesthetists and Non-acute Pain Management*, 1993.

84. McQuay H et al, 'Systematic Review of Outpatient Services for Chronic Pain Control', *Health Technology Assessment*, 1(6), 1997.

85. Everatt R, 'Pain Management', *Nursing Times*, 91:40-1, 1995.

86. Crombie I K and Davies H T O, 'Audit of Outpatients: Entering the Loop', *BMJ*, 302:1437-9, 1991.

87. Davies H T O, Crombie I K & Macrae W A, 'Waiting in Pain', *Anaesthesia*, 49:661-5, 1994.

88. Weir R et al, 'A Profile of Users of Specialty Pain Clinic Services: Predictors of Use and Cost Estimates', *Journal of Clinical Epidemiology*, 45:1399-1415, 1992.

89. Pither C E & Ralphs J A, 'Limiting the Drugs List: Behavioural Treatment', *BMJ*, 306:1687-8, 1993.

90. Irvine D, 'The Performance of Doctors. I: Professionalism and Self-regulation in a Changing World', *BMJ*, 314:1540-2, 1997.

91. Irvine D, 'The Performance of Doctors II: Maintaining Good Practice, Protecting Patients from Poor Performance', *BMJ*, 314:1613-5, 1997.

92. Simpson J & Scott T, 'Beyond the Call of Duty', *Health Service Journal*, 8 May 1997, pp22-5.

93. Calman C, 'The Profession of Medicine', *BMJ*, 309:1140-3, 1994.

94. Abenstein J P & Warner M A, 'Anesthesia Providers, Patient Outcomes, and Costs', *Anesthesia and Analgesia*, 82:1273-83, 1996.

95. Zambricki C S, 'Anesthesia Providers, Patient Outcomes, and Costs': the AANA responds to the Abenstein and Warner article in the June 1996 *Anesthesia and Analgesia, AANA Journal*, 64:413-16, 1996.

96. Reilly C et al, *Professional Roles in Anaesthetics: A Scoping Study*, NHS Executive, Leeds, 1996.

97. NHS Executive, *Good Practice in Operating Theatre Management*, Department of Health.

98. Goddard J M & Pickup S E, 'Postoperative Pain in Children: Combining Audit and A Clinical Nurse Specialist to Improve Management', *Anaesthesia*, 51: 588-90, 1996.

99. Broadway P J & Jones J G, 'A Method of Costing Anaesthetic Practice', *Anaesthesia*, 50:56-63, 1995.

100. Copp L A, 'Pain Coping', in Copp L A (ed), *Perspectives On Pain*: Recent Advances in Nursing, II, Churchill Livingstone, Edinburgh, 1985.

Index References are to paragraph numbers, Boxes and Case Studies